T0192131

Quick
Reference
Dictionary

QRD

FOR GI and
Hepatology

Quick
Reference
Dictionary

FOR GI and
Hepatology

Q
R
D

Edited by

Jonathan M. Fenkel, MD
Assistant Professor of Medicine
Director, Jefferson Hepatitis C Center
Associate Medical Director of Liver Transplantation
Division of Gastroenterology and Hepatology
Thomas Jefferson University Hospital
Philadelphia, Pennsylvania

CRC Press
Taylor & Francis Group
Boca Raton London New York

CRC Press is an imprint of the
Taylor & Francis Group, an **informa** business

First published 2014 by SLACK Incorporated

Published 2024 by CRC Press
2385 NW Executive Center Drive, Suite 320, Boca Raton FL 33431

and by CRC Press
4 Park Square, Milton Park, Abingdon, Oxon, OX14 4RN

CRC Press is an imprint of Taylor & Francis Group, LLC

© 2014 Taylor & Francis Group, LLC

Quick reference dictionary for GI and hepatology / edited by Jonathan M. Fenkel.

p. ; cm.

Includes bibliographical references and index.

ISBN 978-1-61711-019-1 (alk. paper)

I. Fenkel, Jonathan M., 1978- editor.

[DNLM: 1. Gastrointestinal Diseases--Dictionary--English. 2. Gastrointestinal Diseases--Handbooks. 3. Gastroenterology--Dictionary--English. 4. Gastroenterology--Handbooks. 5. Gastrointestinal Tract--Dictionary--English. 6. Gastrointestinal Tract--Handbooks. WI 13]

RC801

616.3'3003--dc23

2014002648

ISBN: 9781617110191 (pbk)
ISBN: 9781003526162 (ebk)

DOI: 10.1201/9781003526162

Dedication

To my late grandfather, Samuel Wisotsky, whose need for physical therapy morphed into this book in a way that you would have to know him to understand.

Contents

Acknowledgments

Thank you to my wife, Michele, for her love, encouragement, and patience. Thank you also to my children, Ezra and Zoe, who missed some quality time with me while I completed this book. I also wish to thank the staff at SLACK Incorporated, and in particular, Carrie Kotlar, for her wise insight, guidance and patience. Furthermore, I couldn't have done this without all of my contributors—thanks for all of your hard work and dedication.

Acknowledgment

About the Editor

Jonathan M. Fenkel, MD is an assistant professor of medicine at Thomas Jefferson University in Philadelphia, Pennsylvania, where he is also Director of the Jefferson Hepatitis C Center and Associate Medical Director of Liver Transplantation. He is board certified in internal medicine, gastroenterology, and transplant hepatology by the American Board of Internal Medicine. Dr. Fenkel graduated cum laude and as a Benjamin Franklin Scholar from the University of Pennsylvania and magna cum laude from Jefferson Medical College, both in Philadelphia, Pennsylvania. He completed his internal medicine residency at the University of Maryland Medical Center in Baltimore, Maryland, and completed fellowships in gastroenterology and transplant hepatology at Thomas Jefferson University in Philadelphia, Pennsylvania.

Dr. Fenkel has been recognized by his peers and trainees as an outstanding educator, including a faculty teaching award in his first year of practice. He has authored more than 40 scientific works, including peer-reviewed journal articles, book chapters, abstracts, and poster presentations. He is a member of the editorial board of the *World Journal of Hepatology*. He has served as an invited peer reviewer for many prestigious journals, including the *Journal of the American Medical Association, Hepatology, Digestive Diseases and Sciences,* and the *Scandinavian Journal of Gastroenterology.*

Contributing Authors

Jennifer S. Au, MD
Fellow
Division of Gastroenterology/
  Hepatology
Scripps Clinic
La Jolla, California

Alia S. Dadabhai, MD
Assistant Professor of
  Medicine
Johns Hopkins University
Division of Digestive
  Diseases
Baltimore, Maryland

Jessica Jackson, MD
Resident
Urology
University of Virginia Health
  System
Charlottesville, Virginia

Annsley Klehr, MEd
Gluten Freedoms, LLC
eat. live. be. gluten free.
www.glutenfreedoms.com

Steven Krawitz, MD
Fellow
Division of Gastroenterology
  and Hepatology
Thomas Jefferson University
  Hospital
Philadelphia, Pennsylvania

Christina Lindenmeyer, MD
Resident
Internal Medicine
Thomas Jefferson University
  Hospital
Philadelphia, Pennsylvania

Aaron Mendelson, MD
Resident
Internal Medicine
Hospital of the University of
  Pennsylvania
Philadelphia, Pennsylvania

Anastasia Shnitser, MD
Assistant Professor
University of South Florida
  School of Medicine
Clinical Gastroenterologist
Lehigh Valley Hospital
Allentown, Pennsylvania

Colin L. Smith, MD
Fellow
Division of Gastroenterology
    and Hepatology
Thomas Jefferson University
    Hospital
Philadelphia, Pennsylvania

Joanna Tolin, MD
Instructor of Clinical
    Medicine
Department of Medicine
Section of Hospital Medicine
Hospital of the University of
    Pennsylvania
Philadelphia, Pennsylvania

Introduction

This easy-to-use quick reference guide is designed to provide convenient, high yield information pertaining to the fields of gastroenterology and hepatology. More than 1100 words and 26 appendices provide up-to-date, clinically relevant definitions and data targeted for trainees in the field of gastroenterology, mid-level practitioners, medical students, industry trainees, and others seeking advancement of their knowledge in digestive diseases.

Jonathan M. Fenkel, MD

abdomen: The anatomical area located between the chest and pelvis, colloquially referred to as the belly or gut. The diaphragm and pelvic bones compose the upper and lower borders, respectively. Classically, it is divided into four quadrants: right upper, right lower, left upper, and left lower.

abdominal girth: The circumference of the abdomen, typically measured at the level of the umbilicus.

abdominal migraine: A disorder of intermittent pain in the abdomen associated with flushing, pallor, nausea, and vomiting that lasts less than 72 hours, with complete resolution of symptoms between attacks. It is most common in children and often lacks a concomitant aura or headache. However, if an aura occurs, symptoms may be prevented by pre-emptive use of triptan-type antimigraine medications.

abdominal pain: Discomfort or distress located in the abdomen. Pain may arise from an organ or disease within the abdomen itself or be referred to the abdomen from another region of the body.

aberrant hepatic artery: A common anatomical variation occurring in approximately 40% of people wherein the hepatic artery origin is from a vessel other than the celiac trunk. The artery can be a replacing artery (one that exists in the absence of a normal hepatic artery) or an accessory artery (one that exists in addition to a normal hepatic artery).

abetalipoproteinemia: An autosomal recessive disorder caused by a mutation in the microsomal triglyercide transfer protein leading to the malabsorption of fats and fat-soluble vitamins secondary to absent apolipoprotein B, an essential component of chylomicrons and very-low-density lipoproteins. Steatorrhea is one of the common presenting signs; *also called* Bassen-Kornzweig syndrome.

abscess: A collection of pus that can occur in any area of the body. It is typically caused by a bacterial infection, which leads to inflammation and swelling. Treatment includes antibiotics, drainage, or both, depending on the location.

absolute risk reduction: An epidemiologic calculation determined by subtracting the experimental group event rate from the control group event rate. For example, if a disease is present in 20% of control subjects but in only 5% of subjects receiving an experimental medication, then the absolute risk reduction would be (20% – 5%) = 15%.

acalculous cholecystitis: An acute inflammatory disease of the gallbladder not caused by gallstone disease that accounts for 10% of all acute cholecystitis cases. The condition is associated with high morbidity and mortality.

acanthosis nigricans: A darkened, hyperpigmented skin discoloration typically involving the intertriginous areas, such as the axilla and groin. Presence of this rash is typically associated with obesity and diabetes mellitus but may also be associated with underlying GI malignancy.

accessory pancreatic duct: Anatomical variant in which a branch duct located off the main pancreatic duct is formed in the head of the pancreas. The accessory duct may drain separately and directly into the duodenum at the minor duodenal papilla; *also called* duct of Santorini.

acetaminophen: A common over-the-counter medication used as an analgesic and for its antipyretic (fever-reducing) properties. Use can cause direct liver damage when more than the recommended daily dosage of 4000 mg is taken or even at therapeutic doses when taken in combination with alcohol or during fasting. The antidote to acetaminophen is N-acetylcysteine, which is available orally or intravenously.

acetylcholine: A neurotransmitter used in the peripheral, central, and autonomic nervous systems.

achalasia: An esophageal motility disorder characterized by aperistalsis, increased resting (basal) tone of the lower esophageal sphincter, and incomplete relaxation of the lower esophageal sphincter during swallowing. Symptoms include progressive dysphagia to liquids and solids, as well as regurgitation of undigested food. There may be progressive dilation of the esophagus above the lower esophageal sphincter, which classically appears like a bird's beak on a barium swallow study. Pathophysiology is thought to involve the loss of inhibitory neurons in the smooth muscle of the distal esophagus.

achlorhydria: Absence of acid production by the gastric parietal cells, which can be a consequence of drug therapy or chronic atrophic gastritis.

acid reflux: *See* gastroesophageal reflux disease.

acinar cell: An exocrine pancreatic cell that secretes digestive enzymes. Cells are arranged in groups called acini that resemble a cluster of grapes. Digestive enzymes are released from the acini and reach the duodenum through a system of pancreatic ducts.

acinar cell carcinoma: A rare neoplasm of the exocrine pancreas that most commonly presents in white men in their fifth or sixth decade. It accounts for 1% to 2% of pancreatic exocrine tumors and is frequently at an advanced stage at the time of diagnosis.

acinarization: Visualization of the pancreatic duct side branches and parenchyma as a result of excessive injection of contrast material into the main pancreatic duct during an endoscopic retrograde cholangiopancreatography (ERCP). It is thought to be a risk factor for post-ERCP pancreatitis due to the hydrostatic pressure caused by overinjection of the contrast material.

acrodermatitis: A rash involving the hands and feet that usually occurs in childhood and can be associated with a febrile illness. It should be distinguished from acrodermatitis enteropathica, which is a distinct entity resulting from impaired absorption of zinc.

acrodermatitis enteropathica: A rare autosomal recessive genetic disorder resulting in defective zinc absorption that is characterized by a pustular rash usually located around the mouth, hands, feet, and anus and is accompanied by diarrhea and alopecia. Symptoms are the same as those that occur in individuals with acquired zinc deficiency. Treatment is the prescription of oral zinc supplementation.

acupuncture: A form of traditional Chinese medicine that is most often used to treat pain. It involves the insertion of very thin needles into strategic places on the skin.

acute appendicitis: Inflammation of the appendix that can be caused by an appendiceal obstruction or infection. It is a common cause of acute abdomen; *see* appendicitis.

acute cholangitis: An infection of the biliary tract usually caused by a biliary obstruction, such as common bile duct stones or strictures. It may result in a clinical syndrome of fever, jaundice, and right upper quadrant abdominal pain (*known as* Charcot's triad). Treatment includes prompt antibiotics and biliary drainage; *also called* ascending cholangitis.

acute cholecystitis: Inflammation of the gallbladder wall. It is usually an infectious complication of cystic duct obstruction caused by gallstones. Diagnosis can be made using an ultrasound, computed tomography (CT) scan, or hydroxyiminodiacetic acid (HIDA) scan.

acute colitis: Inflammation of the wall of the colon that develops over a short period of time. It may be idiopathic, ischemic, infectious, or inflammatory in etiology. Typical symptom presentation includes abdominal pain, diarrhea, and rectal bleeding.

acute fatty liver of pregnancy: Fatty infiltration of liver hepatocytes occurs during pregnancy and may result in liver failure. The disease most commonly presents in the third trimester and usually resolves after delivery. It may be difficult to distinguish from the hemolysis, elevated liver enzymes, and low platelet count (HELLP) syndrome. It is caused by a deficiency of long-chain 3-hydroxyacyl-coenzyme A dehydrogenase (L-CHAD). Symptom presentation includes nausea, vomiting, abdominal pain, and jaundice; blood tests reveal abnormal liver enzymes, hypoglycemia, and coagulopathy; *compare* hemolysis, elevated liver enzymes, and low platelet count (HELLP) syndrome.

acute gastritis: Inflammation of the gastric mucosa occurring over a short period of time. Common causes include infection with *Helicobacter pylori* and exposure to nonsteroidal anti-inflammatory drugs (NSAIDs). Treatment involves removal of inciting causes and cessation of proton pump inhibitors.

acute liver failure: Rapid deterioration of liver function due to severe hepatocyte injury, resulting in coagulopathy (international normalized ratio [INR] ≥1.5) or mental status changes (encephalopathy) in a patient without previously known liver disease. When encephalopathy is present, the liver failure is considered fulminant. Common causes of acute liver failure include viral hepatitis, drug-induced liver injury, and autoimmune hepatitis. A liver transplant is often needed for survival if no reversible cause is identified quickly.

acute pancreatitis: Abrupt onset of inflammation of the pancreas. Common etiologies include alcohol or other drugs or obstruction of the pancreatic duct by gallstones or tumor. It classically presents with epigastric pain radiating to the back and is associated with nausea and vomiting. Severe cases may be associated with multiorgan system failure; *see* Appendix 23.

adenocarcinoma: Cancer of any glandular epithelial tissue. Many GI organs, including the colon, stomach, and esophagus, can develop adenocarcinoma.

adenoma: A benign neoplasm of epithelial cells, with the potential for malignant degeneration into cancer. The colon is the most common site in the GI tract for adenomas.

adenomatous polyp: A benign neoplastic growth originating from glandular epithelial tissue in the GI tract that has the potential for malignant degeneration. Adenomas are the most common type of colonic polyp and are classified based on their size and their macroscopic and microscopic appearance. Larger polyps typically confer the greatest risk of transforming into colon cancer. The number and size of the adenomatous polyps found during a screening colonoscopy determine the interval to the patient's next screening colonoscopy.

adenomatous polyposis coli (APC) gene: A tumor suppressor gene located on chromosome 5 that, when absent or mutated, can be associated with de novo or familial colorectal cancer (CRC) (familial adenomatous polyposis [FAP], attenuated FAP).

adenomyomatosis: A benign condition of the gallbladder characterized by overgrowth of the mucosa, thickening of the muscle layer, and intramural diverticula (called Rokitansky-Aschoff sinuses). Despite its name, no actual adenoma formation occurs and the condition is not thought to be premalignant.

adenopathy: *Another term for* lymphadenopathy.

adenovirus: A double-stranded deoxyribonucleic acid (DNA) virus that commonly causes respiratory illness, such as the common cold or bronchitis. Adenoviruses can also cause a wide range of other illnesses, such as gastroenteritis or neurologic disease. More than 50 types of adenoviruses exisit and can cause human illness.

adhesion: Fibrous tissue located in the abdominal cavity as a result of surgery or an inflammatory disorder. Adhesions are among the most common causes of bowel obstruction.

adventitia: A layer of connective tissue that forms the outermost surface of many organs and blood vessels. In the GI tract, adventitia lines the surface of the organs that lie outside the peritoneal cavity, such as the majority of the esophagus, portions of the colon, and the rectum. Intraperitoneal organs are instead lined by serosa, which is a layer of connective tissue covered by epithelial cells.

afferent loop syndrome: A condition occurring as a result of a gastrojejunostomy in which the upstream bile limb can become acutely or chronically obstructed. A HIDA scan is useful in the diagnosis of this condition.

African iron overload: A tendency to develop increased iron stores, observed in people of southern African descent. It is associated with a polymorhpism in the gene for ferroportin, a transmembrane protein involved in iron transport. It was formerly referred to as Bantu siderosis.

AIDS cholangiopathy: A type of obstructive biliary disease seen in patients with acquired immune deficiency syndrome (AIDS) caused by opportunistic infections that results in stricturing of the biliary tree. The most common pathogen is *Cryptosporidium parvum.*

Alagille syndrome: An inherited autosomal dominant condition characterized by a paucity of bile ducts resulting in cholestatic liver disease. It is caused by mutations in the Jagged1 gene on chromosome 20 and, to a lesser extent, the Notch2 gene. It is also associated with cardiac, skeletal, renal, and ocular abnormalities; *also called* Alagille-Watson syndrome.

Alagille-Watson syndrome: *Another term for* Alagille syndrome.

alanine aminotransferase (ALT): An enzyme produced mainly in the liver that catalyzes a reversible reaction involving the transfer of an amino group to form pyruvate and glutamate. Acute hepatitis or ongoing hepatocyte injury often results in elevated blood levels; *also called* serum glutamic pyruvic transaminase.

albumin: Synthesized by the liver, it is the most abundant protein found in plasma and functions to maintain oncotic pressure, as well as transport different molecules in the bloodstream. Low levels of albumin (hypoalbuminemia) are often caused by chronic liver disease or cirrhosis.

alcoholic hepatitis: Acute alcohol-induced injury to the liver that is classically characterized by the rapid onset of jaundice, fever, elevated transaminase levels, and pathologic findings of swollen (ballooned) hepatocytes with inclusion bodies (*known as* Mallory bodies), macrovesicular fat (steatosis), and polymorphonuclear infiltrate. Severe cases can result in liver failure and death; *see* Appendix 5.

alkaline phosphatase: An enzyme found in all tissues that functions to cleave phosphate groups from many types of molecules in an alkaline environment. The liver, bile ducts, bone, and small intestine have high levels of this enzyme. Elevated blood levels may suggest injury to any of those tissues. Alkaline phosphatase of liver and bile duct origins can be distinguished from that of bone and small bowel through laboratory testing.

aloe vera: A species of the aloe plant whose leaves produce a thick gel that can be used as a topical emollient to soothe skin. The inner lining of the plant's leaves has laxative properties and can be found in some over-the-counter laxatives.

alpha fetoprotein: A plasma protein normally produced by the yolk sac and liver during fetal development. The function of circulating levels in adults is unknown. Elevated levels may occur in germ cell tumors, hepatocellular carcinoma, and ataxia telangiectasia.

alpha-1 antitrypsin deficiency: An inherited disorder characterized by lung (early emphysema) and liver disease (cirrhosis) as a result of a serum deficiency and impaired hepatic clearance of the protein alpha-1 antitrypsin, an antagonistic enzyme to neutrophil elastase. The phenotype most associated with liver disease is ZZ, although heterozygotes may still be at risk of chronic liver disease.

amebiasis: A parasitic disease of the GI tract caused by *Entamoeba histolytica* that is spread by fecal-oral transmission. The parasites most frequently invade the right colon. Antiparasitic agents, including metronidazole and paromomycin, are used in treatment.

amebic abscess: A complication of intestinal infection with the parasite *E histolytica,* whereby the parasites invade the splanchnic blood vessels and spread to the liver where they form collections of pus. Metronidizole is a common antibiotic used in treatment.

amebic colitis: A complication of infection with the parasite *E histolytica.* The parasites invade the colonic epithelium and burrow through to the submucosa, causing colonic inflammation, which can progress to toxic megacolon if untreated.

American Association for the Study of Liver Diseases (AASLD): Founded in 1950, the AASLD is an international society that aims to "advance the science and practice of hepatology, liver transplantation, and hepatobiliary surgery, thereby promoting liver health and optimal care of patients with liver and biliary tract diseases." Website: www.aasld.org

American College of Gastroenterology (ACG): Founded in 1932, the ACG is an international organization with more than 12,000 members that aims to "advance the medical treatment and scientific study of GI disorders." Website: www.gi.org

American Gastroenterological Association (AGA): Founded in 1897, the AGA is an international organization with more than 17,000 members that aims "[t]o advance the science and practice of gastroenterology." Website: www.gastro.org

American Society for Gastrointestinal Endoscopy (ASGE): Founded in 1941, the ASGE is an international society with more than 12,000 members dedicated to "advancing patient care and digestive health by promoting excellence and innovation in GI endoscopy." Website: www.asge.org

amine precursor uptake and decarboxylation (APUD) cell: Peptide hormone-secreting cells of the endocrine system located throughout the GI system and in other endocrine organs throughout the body.

aminosalicylates: Anti-inflammatory medications containing 5-aminosalicylic acid that are used in the treatment of many diseases, including inflammatory bowel disease (IBD). There are several types of aminosalicylates, with formulations designed for absorbtion in different portions of the GI tract to treat patients with disease confined to certain areas.

ambulatory pH monitoring: A technique used to measure the amount and timing of acid refluxed from the stomach into the esophagus. A small device is placed in the esophagus to record acid exposure over 24 to 48 hours. The information can then be transmitted wirelessly or directly to a receiving device carried by the patient. It is considered the gold standard for diagnosising acid reflux.

ampulla of Vater: The union of the main pancreatic duct and common bile duct at the major duodenal papilla in the second portion of the duodenum. It was named for 18th century German anatomist Abraham Vater; *also called* the hepatopancreatic ampulla.

ampullary cancer: A malignant tumor present at the ampulla of Vater. Most commonly, it is an adenocarcionma that can present as a biliary obstruction, abdominal pain, jaundice, or unintentional weight loss.

Amsterdam criteria: A set of criteria established to identify patients or families at risk for Lynch syndrome (*also known as* hereditary nonpolyposis colon cancer). To fulfill the criteria, a patient must have at least 3 relatives with colon cancer, of which at least one is a first-degree relative of the other two; the cases must occur over at least two generations; and one must be diagnosed before age 50 years; *see also* Lynch syndrome.

amylase: An enzyme secreted by the salivary glands and pancreas that breaks down and digests carbohydrates. Elevated blood levels of amylase can be seen in patients with pancreatitis.

amyloidosis: A broad term referring to the abnormal deposition of fibrils of proteins, usually those found in plasma, into extracellular tissues. Amyloidosis may be primary (*known as* AL amyloidosis) or secondary (*known as* AA amyloidosis). In AL amyloidosis, the deposited protein is derived from immunoglobulin light chains. AA amyloidosis results from deposition of fragments of serum amyloid A, which is an acute phase reactant released in response to ongoing inflammation from chronic diseases.

anal canal: The 3- to 4-cm long tubular structure that connects the rectum to the opening of the anus.

anal fissure: A superficial tear in the mucosa of the anal canal often caused by constipation with straining, usually resulting in painful defecation with blood spotting. Chronic fissures are more commonly found in the posterior aspect of the anal canal. Medical treatments include stool softeners, topical nitroglycerin, or botox to prevent anal spasm.

anal papilla: Raised tooth-like tissue projections at the anus extending into the rectum, which may become hypertrophied by inflammation or fibrosis. Often referred to as anal skin tags when hypertrophied.

anal stenosis: Abnormal narrowing of the anal canal. Common causes include congenital anomaly, scarring from surgical procedures (such as hemorrhoidectomy), or inflammatory disease (such as Crohn's disease).

anemia: A decrease in hemoglobin with a resultant decrease in the oxygen-carrying capacity of the blood. It can be caused by decreased production of red blood cells by the bone marrow, by abnormal destruction of red cells such as in hemolytic anemia, or from blood loss due to acute or chronic bleeding, often originating from the GI tract.

angiodypslasia: *Another term for* angioectasia.

angiodysplasias: *See* arteriovenous malformation.

angioectasia: A vascular abnormality in which there is dilation of a small blood vessel near the mucosal surface of an organ. These may be seen anywhere in the GI tract and can cause sporadic bleeding. Endoscopic treatment with argon plasma coagulation, bipolar electrocautery, or endoclips is the first-line treatment; *also called* angiodypslasia.

angioectasias: *See* arteriovenous malformation.

angular cheilitis: The development of cracks, sores, or ulcers at the corners of the mouth that are often due to a fungal infection but can be seen in individuals with severe vitamin deficiencies or severely chapped lips; *also called* perleche.

anismus: A spasm-like defecatory difficulty caused by functional obstruction due to malfunction of the external anal sphincter or puborectalis muscle. It is more common in women than men; *also called* spastic pelvic floor syndrome.

anomalous pancreaticobiliary ductal union: A condition in which the main pancreatic duct and the common bile duct merge to form a common channel outside of the duodenum that is more than 15 mm in length. It may be associated with a higher lifetime risk of gallbladder cancer.

anorectal manometry: A test that measures pressures of the anal sphincter muscles and is used to evaluate patients who have problems with defecation, including constipation and fecal incontinence. A small tube with a balloon is inserted into the rectum and used to measure pressures generated by the anal sphincters to determine the etiology of a defecation disorder.

anorectum: The anatomic area between the dentate line and the anal verge.

anorexia: A lack of appetite or inability to eat.

anorexia nervosa: An eating disorder characterized by a severe restriction of oral intake, an irrational fear of gaining weight, excessive weight loss, and a distorted body perception. It is most common in young women. Refeeding syndrome may occur in patients who abruptly resume eating, so careful monitoring for this condition is imperative.

antacid: A medication used to counteract the symptoms of heartburn. It typically refers to calcium-based, over-the-counter medications but also includes histamine-receptor antagonists and proton pump inhibitors.

anti-diarrheal: A medication used to counteract the symptom of diarrhea.

anti-emetic: A medication used to counteract the symptom of nausea.

anti-liver cytosol 1 (Anti-LC1) antibody: A serologic marker associated with type 2 autoimmune hepatitis primarily found in patients younger than 20 years and rare in patients older than 40 years.

anti-liver kidney microsomal (Anti-LKM) antibody: A serologic marker associated with type 2 autoimmune hepatitis found in approximately 4% of American adults with autoimmune hepatitis.

antimitochondrial antibody (AMA): A serologic marker found in 95% of patients with primary biliary cirrhosis. It can also be found in 5% to 20% of patients with autoimmune hepatitis and is 95% sensitive and 98% specific for primary biliary cirrhosis.

antinuclear antibody (ANA): A serologic marker for systemic or organ-specific autoimmune disease and the most common circulating autoantibody in type 1 autoimmune hepatitis. In most laboratories, titers greater than 1:80 are considered positive in adults.

antireflux surgery: Surgical management for severe reflux disease (including refractory esophagitis), persistent reflux symptoms despite acid suppression, or extra-esophageal manifestations of acid reflux, such as asthma or laryngeal esophageal reflux disease. This phrase typically refers to a fundoplication, where the lower esophageal sphincter is reinforced by wrapping part of the stomach around it. Common variations of fundoplication include Nissen (360 degree), Toupet (270 degree), and Dor (180 degree).

anti-*Saccharomyces cerevisiae* antibody (ASCA): Serologic marker often associated with Crohn's disease found in 40% to 80% of patients with ileocecal involvement and most often absent in patients with ulcerative colitis.

anti-smooth muscle antibody (anti-SMA): Serologic marker found in 87% of cases of type 1 autoimmune hepatitis that is more specific, but less prevalent than ANA.

anti-soluble liver antigen (Anti-SLA): Serologic marker associated with type 1 autoimmune hepatitis found in 10% to 30% of adult patients but more common in children with type 1 and type 2 autoimmune hepatitis.

antroduodenal manometry: A catheter-based test that records changes in intraluminal pressure during various periods of GI motility, including the contractile activity of the distal stomach and proximal small bowel during fasting, after eating, and while sleeping. Recordings may last from 5 hours (stationary study) to 24 hours (ambulatory study), and it is primarily used to evaluate patients for dyspepsia, gastroparesis, or chronic intestinal pseudo-obstruction with unexplained upper GI symptoms (eg, nausea, vomiting).

antrum: Distal part of the stomach, proximal to the pyloric sphincter. It is the primary location of gastrin-producing G cells (responsible for stimulating acid production) and somatostatin-producing D cells (responsible for downregulating or shutting off acid secretion).

aortoenteric fistula: Abnormal connection between the abdominal aorta or an abdominal aortic graft and a portion of the bowel. The most common location is the fourth portion of the duodenum. It classically presents with a herald GI bleed, a self-limited severe bleeding episode, which is then followed by life-threatening, massive GI bleeding.

appendectomy: Surgical removal of the appendix. It can be performed using an open or laparoscopic procedure or via natural orifice transluminal endoscopic surgery (NOTES). It is one of the most common surgical procedures performed around the world.

appendiceal adenocarcinoma: A rare form of cancer arising from the appendix that can have variable clinical presentations, including acute appendicitis, abdominal pain, abdominal mass, or ascites. It exists in three histologic variants: mucinous type, intestinal or colonic type, and signet ring cell adenocarcinoma. Treatment for early disease is a right hemicolectomy. Prognosis is based on histological variant with a 5-year survival rate of more than 80% for treated mucinous type and less than 35% for treated signet ring variant.

appendiceal carcinoid: A neuroendocrine tumor of the appendix that can secrete serotonin, norepinephrine, dopamine, and other vasoactive substances. Typically, these are located in the distal one-third of the appendix, and 90% are metastatic at the time of presentation (usually the liver). Octreoscan is the most sensitive study for diagnosis and staging. Treatment is based on tumor size, with tumors smaller than 2 cm usually managed by appendectomy alone, whereas larger tumors are treated with right hemicolectomy.

appendiceal orifice: An endoscopically indentified landmark located in the cecum that indicates the location of the appendix and appears as a puckered-like area at the cecal base. Documentation of this landmark is considered standard during a colonoscopy.

appendicitis: Inflammation of the appendix typically presenting as acute onset of abdominal pain in the epigastrium and then radiating to the right lower quadrant (at McBurney's point). It can also be chronic in duration.

appendix (vermiform appendix): A blind-ended tube at the base of the cecum without a clearly understood function.

apthous ulcer: A type of ulcer found on the mucous membranes. Many potential causes exist, including autoimmune diseases, infections, drugs, trauma, medications, nutritional deficiencies, and poor oral care.

argon plasma coagulation (APC): The use of jet-ionized argon gas (plasma) to control mucosal bleeding. Lesions in the GI tract are often amenable to APC via endoscopy and include angiodysplasias or arteriovenous malformations, gastric antral vascular ectasia, radiation proctitis, esophageal cancer, and postpolypectomy bleeding.

arteriovenous malformation (AVM): A congenital vascular abnormality connecting the venous and arterial system and bypassing the capillary tract. AVMs are asymptomatic 88% of the time but can also cause bleeding if located in the GI tract; *also called* angioectasias or angiodysplasias in the GI tract. AVMs can be found anywhere in the body but are typically in one isolated organ system. They can also be associated with multiorgan diseases, such as Von Hippel-Lindau disease or hereditary hemorrhagic telangectasias.

Ascaris lumbricoides: A roundworm parasite and the most common human helminthic infection worldwide. Infection is usually asymptomatic but can cause an intestinal obstruction if there is a large worm burden, abdominal pain, or biliary obstruction. Albendazole is used for treatment. Nitazoxanide, ivermectin, and mebendazole are alternative treatment regimens.

ascending cholangitis: *Another term for* acute cholangitis.

ascending colon: Right side of the colon extending from the cecum to the hepatic flexure.

ascites: Fluid accumulation in the peritoneal cavity resulting from portal hypertension, malignancy, infection, heart failure, nephrotic syndrome, or protein deficiency. Paracentesis and calculation of the serum ascites albumin gradient can be used to identify the cause of the ascites.

aspartate aminotransferase (AST): An enzyme that catalyzes a reversible reaction involving the transfer of an α-amino group between aspartate and glutamate. It is located in the liver primarily but is also present in the heart, skeletal muscle, kidneys, brain, and red blood cells. Elevated serum levels suggest injury to any of these organ systems but are most commonly associated with liver injury; *also called* serum glutamic oxaloacetic transaminase.

aspiration: 1. Removal of fluid from a collection of fluid using a needle or catheter. 2. The unintentional inhalation of food or fluid into the respiratory system that may precipitate pneumonitis or pneumonia.

aspiration pneumonia: Inflammation, infection, or both of the bronchial tree or lung parenchyma after oral or gastric contents are introduced into the pulmonary system via aspiration. Predispoing conditions include recent stroke, lingering effects of anesthesia, and achalasia. Treatment is antibiotics, correction of predisposing situations, and supportive care.

asterixis: Involuntary flapping motion of an outstretched, dorsiflexed hand that can be a sign of decompensated liver disease, specifically hepatic encephalopathy. It can also be seen in uremic renal failure, lithium toxicity, subthalamic infarct, and severe electrolyte disturbances.

atrophic gastritis: Inflammation of the stomach mucosa leading to loss of gastric glandular cells and their secretion of hydrochloric acid, pepsin, and intrinsic factor resulting in dyspepsia, digestive difficulties, vitamin B_{12} deficiency, and pernicious anemia. This condition can be incited by *H pylori* infection or autoimmunity. It is further differentiated into Type A (body/fundus of the stomach) and the more common Type B (antrum-central stomach).

attenuated familial adenomatous polyposis (AFAP): A form of FAP characterized by fewer than 100 colorectal adenomas. It is usually limited to the right side of the colon and has a less aggressive onset than classic FAP and a more aggressive onset than colorectal carcinoma. It is caused by a mutation in the adenomatous polyposis coli gene. Diagnosis requires genetic testing due to a reduced number of polyps compared with standard FAP.

autoimmune cholangiopathy: An overlap syndrome between autoimmune hepatitis, sclerosing cholangitis, and primary biliary cirrhosis that is often responsive to steroids. It may have the clinical or biochemical features of cholestasis, a high titer antinuclear antibody, a negative antimitochondrial antibody, and an elevated immunoglobulin G.

autoimmune enteropathy: Rare autoimmune disease directed at gut epithelial cell antibodies and related to other autoimmune diseases in 80% of cases. Small intestinal histopathologic findings are subtotal villous atrophy and lymphoplasmacytic infiltration in the lamina propria with relatively few surface intraepithelial lymphocytes. Serum anti-enteroctye antibodies are often present.

autoimmune gastritis: An autosomal dominant disorder that causes injury to the gastric mucosa (typically body and fundus) and is marked by an immune response against the parietal cells and an intrinsic factor leading to profound hypochlorhydria and elevated gastrin levels. The affected patients often develop pernicious anemia from vitamin B_{12} malabsorption. Elevated gastrin levels lead to increased enterochromaffin cells and can predispose individuals to malignant transformation.

autoimmune hepatitis: A disorder caused by autoimmune antibodies directed toward the liver that can result in inflammation and cirrhosis. Type 1, or classic autoimmune hepatitis, is characterized by circulating antibodies to nuclei (ANA), smooth muscle (ASMA), or both; type 2 is characterized by the presence of anti-LKM or anti-LC1. Elevated gamma globulins may also be present. Steroids or immunomodulators are usually used for treatment. Liver transplantation may be necessary in acute or refractory cases; *also called* lupoid hepatitis; *see* Appendix 6.

autoimmune pancreatitis: A rare disorder of pancreatic inflammation characterized by immune-mediated lymphocytoplasmic infiltration of the pancreas. Elevated serum IgG4 levels are the hallmark of the disease. It may be indistinguishable from pancreatic cancer at presentation. An enlarged, sausage-shaped pancreas with diffuse narrowing of the main pancreatic duct is classically found on cross-sectional imaging. The condition is usually responsive to treatment with corticosteroids, but ERCP may be needed to manage complications of the disorder.

B

bacillary angiomatosis: Cutaneous nodules and papules or sub-cutaneous ulcerations caused by neovascular proliferation secondary to *Bartonella henselae* or *B quintana* infection. It is most often seen in patients with AIDS or those who are otherwise immunocompromised. It can also form painful lytic bone lesions. Treatment is with erythromycin or doxycycline.

Bacillus cereus: A spore-forming, gram-positive bacillus that causes food poisoning and is often observed after eating reheated rice. Severe self-limited nausea and vomiting occur within 2 to 3 hours after infection and last 8 to 10 hours. The bacteria can also produce an enterotoxin, leading to self-limited watery diarrhea and abdominal cramps beginning within 6 to 12 hours and lasting up to 24 hours.

bacteremia: The presence of bacteria in the blood. Blood cultures are used for diagnosis. Treatment requires intravenous antibiotics and investigation into the source.

bacterial overgrowth: *See* small bowel bacterial overgrowth.

balloon dilation: An endoscopic technique used to open narrowed portions of the esophagus or intestines with a through-the-scope balloon. It is most commonly used for strictures occurring from peptic ulcer disease or those that occur postoperatively.

balloon dilator: A device that enables the endoscopist to open a narrowed area of the GI tract. A deflated balloon is passed through an endoscope to the area of concern. It is then inflated using radial force to mechanically open the lumen.

Fenkel JM, ed.
Quick Reference Dictionary for GI and Hepatology (pp 18-26).
© 2014 Taylor & Francis Group.

balloon expulsion test: A procedure used to help determine the cause of chronic constipation in which a balloon is placed in the patient's rectum and then inflated with water. If the patient is unable to expel the inflated balloon, pelvic floor dysfunction may be the cause of constipation.

balloon-occluded retrograde transvenous obliteration (BORTO/ BRTO): A minimally invasive procedure performed by interventional radiologists for the treatment of gastric varices in patients with a spontaneous portosystemic (splenorenal or gastrorenal) shunt as an alternative to a transjugular intrahepatic portosystemic shunt. A balloon is passed over a wire through the femoral vein and shunt and then passed directly into the varices. The balloon is first inflated to occlude the varices, and then a sclerosing agent is injected to prevent them from reopening. This procedure can increase the risk of future formation of esophageal varices and surveillance is recommended.

band ligation: *See* variceal band ligation.

Bannayan-Ruvalcaba-Riley syndrome: An autosomal dominant genetic disorder characterized by hamartomatous polyps in the GI tract, macrocephaly, lipomas, and café au lait spots in the genital region. Sporadic cases may also occur, although this condition is one of the phosphatase and tensin homolog (PTEN) germline mutation-associated hamartoma tumor syndromes (PHTS).

Bantu siderosis: *See* African iron overload.

barium defecography: A radiographic test used to evaluate the causes of constipation or fecal incontinence in which barium is introduced into the rectum and the patient is then asked to try to move his or her bowels while radiographs are taken; *also called* evacuation proctography.

barium enema: A radiographic study used to evaluate the anatomy of the colon in which either barium with air (double-contrast study) or barium alone (single-contrast study) is introduced into the rectum. A radiologist then directs radiographs at the patient's pelvis, which allows the barium to be visualized. It can be useful in the diagnosis of diverticulosis, large polyps, masses, strictures, or inflammatory changes and can be used for the diagnosis and treatment of intussusception.

barium swallow: This study is used to evaluate the esophagus, stomach, and duodenum. The patient drinks barium and radiographs are taken to study its movement down the GI tract. This test is used primarily for the evaluation of dysphagia; *also called* an upper GI series.

Barrett's esophagus: A histologic diagnosis defined as intestinal metaplasia of the esophagus or a change in the normally squamous epithelium found in the esophagus to secretory epithelium usually only found in the small intestines as a result of chronic exposure to acid. Ten percent of cases can progress to dysplasia and less than 1% progress to esophageal adenocarcionma.

BARRX ablation: A specialized endoscopic technique used in the treatment of dysplastic Barrett's esophagus to prevent its progression to cancer by directing a focal source of energy toward the abnormal tissue. BARRX ablation can be deployed using a 90- or 360-degree device attached to the end of the endoscope; *also called* HALO ablation; *see* radiofrequency ablation.

Bartonella henselae: A gram-negative bacillus known for causing cat-scratch disease, as well as bacillary angiomatosis. It can also cause bloody cysts to form in the liver, a rare entity known as peliosis hepatis; *see also* bacillary angiomatosis.

basal acid output: The minimum amount of gastric acid secreted by an individual under normal conditions.

Bassen-Kornzweig syndrome: *Another term for* abetalipoproteinemia.

Behçet's syndrome: A disease characterized by recurrent painful oral and genital ulcers, eye inflammation, and skin lesions. The GI tract can be involved as well, leading to mucosal ulcerations that may mimic Crohn's disease.

benign recurrent intrahepatic cholestasis: An autosomal recessive disorder that can begin in childhood and is characterized by recurrent elevations in liver enzymes and associated itching and jaundice. This condition is not thought to be associated with end-stage liver disease. Symptomatic management is recommended.

bentiromide test: A type of pancreatic function test for exocrine pancreatic insufficiency. Bentiromide is ingested and degraded by chymotrypsin, an enzyme secreted by the pancreas. Its metabolite, para-aminobenzoic acid (PABA), is excreted in the urine. Low urinary levels of PABA indicate that significant pancreatic function has been lost.

beriberi: Clinical syndrome associated with thiamine deficiency that occurs most often in alcoholics or malnourished patients. Dry beriberi is associated with bilateral peripheral neuropathy, leading to sensory and motor deficits. Wet beriberi additionally causes congestive heart failure. Patients with either form respond dramatically after thiamine is reintroduced to his or her diet, with symptomatic improvement in hours to days.

Bernstein test: A test used to diagnose gastroesophageal reflux in which acid is purposefully ingested to reproduce the symptoms of heartburn. If a patient claims that this test reproduces their discomfort, it is considered positive. This is rarely done now secondary to low patient tolerance.

beta blocker(s): Medications that antagonize sympathetic postganglionic beta-1 or beta-2 receptors. Commonly used in the management of hypertension, congestive heart failure, myocardial infarction, and glaucoma. Within gastroenterology, betablockers are used to prevent variceal hemorrhage in patients with portal hypertension.

Bethesda guidelines (criteria): Revised in 2004, these criteria aim to help determine who should undergo genetic testing for hereditary nonpolyposis colon cancer (HNPCC). Meeting any of the following 5 criteria warrant testing: (1) CRC diagnosed before age 50 years; (2) CRC diagnosed simultaneously with an HNPCC-associated malignancy (ie, uterine, ovarian, gastric); (3) CRC diagnosed before age 60 years with high microsatellite instability; (4) CRC diagnosed in one or more first-degree relatives who also have a HNPCC-related malignancy, with one cancer diagnosed before age 50 years; (5) CRC diagnosed in 2 or more first- or second-degree relatives with HNPCC-related malignancy, regardless of their age.

bezoar: A solid mass that accumulates in the GI tract secondary to swallowing specific undigestable items. It is most often found in the stomach. Some examples include masses made of swallowed hair (trichobezoars) or vegetable fibers (phytobezoars). It often requires endoscopy or surgery for removal.

BICAP: A probe that is passed through an endoscope and applies bipolar electrocautery for cauterization of bleeding lesions.

Bier spots: Small, flat, hypopigmented patches on the extremities that can be associated with liver disease.

bile acid reflux: The condition in which bile moves backward from the duodenum into the stomach and esophagus, predisposing individuals to gastritis and esophagitis.

bile acid transporter: An enzyme required to help bile acids in the terminal ileum enter the enterohepatic circulation.

bile duct: A hollow passage that enables bile to move from the liver and gallbladder into the duodenum.

bile ductular proliferation: Increased number of bile ductules on liver biopsy that occurs in the setting of biliary obstruction, primary biliary cirrhosis, or primary sclerosing cholangitis.

biliary atresia: A congenital disorder in which the bile ducts end abruptly without properly connecting to the duodenum, leading to jaundice and progressive liver failure within the first few months of life. Surgery to connect the biliary system to the intestine (*see* Kasai procedure) is life saving, but most patients will ultimately require liver transplantation.

biliary colic: Post prandial abdominal pain or discomfort associated with the presence of cholelithiasis (gallstones). Consuming high fat foods may increase the likelihood of biliary colic. Treatment is with dietary modification, ursodiol, or cholecystectomy.

biliary dyskinesia: Dysfunction of bile acid movement from the ducts into the duodenum, which can be due to any problem resulting in impaired motility or increased pressure at the sphincter of Oddi. Clinically, this causes pain that resembles biliary colic. Treatment aims at increasing transit time through the bile ducts through use of anticholinergic medication or by performing a biliary sphincterotomy.

biliary manometry: A test that helps diagnose biliary dyskinesia or sphincter of Oddi dysfunction. During an ERCP, a small tube is passed from the duodenum into the sphincter of Oddi to obtain pressure measurements; *see* Appendix 25.

biliary obstruction: Physical impedance of bile flow from the liver into the duodenum that can be intrahepatic or extrahepatic in nature. Common etiologies include choledocholithiasis, pancreatic head mass, and biliary strictures. Treatment aims to relieve the obstruction using endoscopic, percutaneous, or surgical therapy.

biliary stenosis: *Another term for* biliary stricture.

biliary stricture: Benign or malignant narrowing of the bile duct. Benign strictures are most often the result of surgery, often as a complication of cholecystectomy. Malignant strictures are due to a tumor located within the bile duct, ampulla, duodenum, or pancreatic head. Endoscopic or surgical treatment is used to dilate, remove, or bypass a strictured segment; *also called* biliary stenosis.

biliary tree: Refers to the bile duct system in its entirety.

bilirubin: A yellowish-colored breakdown product of heme catabolism and a component of bile. Jaundice results when it accumulates at high levels in the blood.

Billroth I: A surgical operation used to treat disorders of the stomach, including ulcers and cancers. The antrum of the stomach is resected, and the remaining parts of the stomach are connected to the duodenum to preserve continuity of the GI tract; *also called* gastroduodenostomy.

Billroth II: A surgical operation to correct stomach disorders that is an alternative to the Billroth I. In this procedure, the antrum is resected and the remaining parts of the stomach are connected to the jejunum, leaving two limbs (efferent and afferent) exiting the stomach. It is a type of gastrojejunostomy.

biofeedback therapy: A type of behavioral therapy designed to enable patients to take control of physiologic processes of which they may not be consciously aware. Within the field of gastroenterology, this technique is used to teach patients with pelvic floor dysfunction or fecal incontinence how to regain control of their anal sphincters.

biopsy: A sample obtained from an organ or tissue during a procedure. For example, during an upper endoscopy, a small forceps can be passed through the working channel of the scope to retrieve a tissue sample from the stomach to evaluate for *H pylori* infection.

biotin: A water-soluble vitamin required for several metabolic processes, including fatty acid synthesis, gluconeogenesis, and amino acid breakdown. Deficiency is rare but can be seen in individuals who consume only egg whites. Symptoms of deficiency include GI upset, rash, scaly skin, hair loss, and mental status changes.

bipolar coagulation: A device that sends an electric current from an electrode into tissue, generating a localized area of energy. It can be used to cut through tissue during surgery or to cauterize a bleeding vessel; *see also* BICAP.

bland embolization: A procedure performed by interventional radiologists for the treatment of liver cancer or for arterial bleeding. Using a femoral artery approach, the desired location is accessed and particulate matter is injected into the tumor-feeding vessel or bleeding artery to cut off its blood supply. Bland embolization is performed without any concurrent chemotherapy. If chemotherapy is added, the procedure is called chemoembolization.

blinded: A research methodology in which patients, researchers, or both are unaware as to which intervention the patient has been randomized. Single-blinded (one party unaware) or double-blinded (both parties unaware) studies can be performed. Blinding helps decrease the placebo effect and observer bias.

blue rubber bleb nevus syndrome: A disorder that causes patients to develop multiple bluish-colored vascular malformations on their skin and internal organs, particularly in the GI tract. It is a rare cause of GI bleeding, intussusception, and anemia.

body mass index (BMI): A calculation used to quantify a patient's degree of obesity. BMI is measured as weight/(height)^2. Categories of BMI are as follows: underweight (BMI lower than 18.5 kg/m^2), normal (BMI between 18.5 and 24.9 kg/m^2), overweight (BMI between 25 and 29.9 kg/m^2), and obese (BMI higher than 30 kg/m^2).

bone densitometry: A radiographic test that measures bone density and is designed to identify patients with osteopenia or osteoporosis.

Borchardt's triad: A triad of symptoms that can be seen in patients with gastric volvulus: acute epigastric abdominal pain, retching without vomiting, and an inability to pass a nasogastric tube.

Boswellia serrata: An Ayurvedic medication used for arthritis and inflammatory conditions, including IBD.

botulinum toxin (BOTOX) therapy: A medical formulation derived from a toxin produced by *Clostridium botulinum* that causes muscle paralysis and relaxation. Within gastroenterology, BOTOX can be directly injected through the endoscope to relax various smooth muscles of the GI tract, including the lower esophageal sphincter (in achalasia) and the pylorus (in gastroparesis).

bougienage: A method used to dilate the lumen of a hollow organ, most often the esophagus, by using cylindrically shaped tubes called bougies.

Bouveret's syndrome: Gastric outlet obstruction caused by a large gallstone impacting itself within the duodenum, preceded by a cholecystoduodenal or cholecystogastric fistula.

bowel obstruction: Occurs when food cannot properly travel through the intestines secondary to either a physical impedance or a lack of motility in the GI tract, leading to abdominal pain, nausea, and vomiting. Common causes include adhesions, hernias, and tumors.

bowel preparation: A regimen of laxatives to cleanse the colon of fecal matter prior to colonoscopy that aids in the visualization of the colon. The quality of a colonoscopy is largely attributable to the quality of the bowel preparation. It can also decrease risk of infection during bowel surgery.

bravo pH monitor: *See* wireless pH monitor.

breath test: A noninvasive technique for diagnosing many GI disorders, including small bowel bacterial overgrowth, *H pylori* infection, and food intolerances. Patients ingest a compound that has a characteristic gaseous signature as measured in the patient's breath.

bridging fibrosis: *See* septal fibrosis.

bronze diabetes: Describes a clinical picture associated with hemo-chromatosis, wherein iron deposition in the liver and pancreas can cause jaundice and diabetes mellitus.

Brunner's gland hyperplasia: Benign growth found in the duo-denum (usually bulb) using endoscopy that is characterized by an increased number of Brunner's glands (glands that normally secrete alkaline mucus into the GI tract). This is usually an incidental finding; however, case reports exist of this condition causing pain, intestinal obstruction, and GI bleeding.

brush cytology: A technique for the acquisition of cellular material to evaluate for infection or malignancy during endoscopy using a thin brush through the endoscope.

Budd-Chiari syndrome: Hepatic venous outflow obstruction, clas-sically caused by thrombosis of the hepatic vein in a hypercoag-ulable patient. Patients present with right upper quadrant pain, variceal bleeding, or abdominal distention, with ascites, jaun-dice, and hepatomegaly detected on examination. Treatment includes anticoagulation, symptom control with paracentesis or endoscopy, transjugular intrahepatic portosystemic shunt, or liver transplantation.

bullous pemphigoid: An autoimmune skin disorder that causes tense, subepidermal blisters to form. Blisters can sometimes involve the mouth, causing dysphagia. Treatment includes steroids, which may predispose patients to peptic ulcer disease.

buried bumper syndrome: A rare complication of percutaneous gastrostomy tube placement when the inside bumper erodes into or through the gastric wall, usually the result of pulling the tube too tightly from the skin. It can present as bleeding after the procedure, pain, or inability to tolerate tube feeds and requires replacement of the tube for treatment.

Byler's disease: *Another term for* PFIC 1; *see* progressive familial intrahepatic cholestasis.

C

C13 urea breath test: A test used in the diagnosis of *H pylori* infection that takes advantage of the fact that *H pylori* can metabolize urea into carbon dioxide and ammonium. A compound containing urea is attached to a radiologic tracer, C13, which is then ingested. If *H pylori* is present in the stomach, the compound is metabolized and releases radiolabeled carbon dioxide, which can be measured in the patient's breath.

C14 urea breath test: A test also used in diagnosis of *H pylori* infection that works exactly the same as the C13 urea breath test but makes use of a radioactive isotope. Although the radiation risk is minimal, some physicians prefer the C13 urea breath test, especially if the patient is pregnant.

C282Y gene: A specific mutation found in the HFE gene located on chromosome 6 that leads to the autosomal recessive disorder hereditary hemochromatosis.

calcineurin inhibitor: A medication that inhibits the actions of calcineurin, a protein involved in the biochemical pathway needed to create interleukin-2 (IL-2), an important cytokine involved in activating the immune system. Drugs included in this family are cyclosporine and tacrolimus. It is often used in patients after a solid-organ transplant to prevent rejection.

calcineurin pathway: A common target of immunosuppression. After activation, the T-cell receptor complex stimulates calcium-dependent calcineurin by combining with inositol triphosphate and immunophilin. This complex dephosphorylates the nuclear factor of activated T-cells (or NF-AT), which migrates to the nucleus and drives transcription of cytokines, particularly IL-2. The immunosuppressive medications tacrolimus and cyclosporine target this pathway; *see* Appendix 7.

Fenkel JM, ed.
Quick Reference Dictionary for GI and Hepatology (pp 27-48).
© 2014 Taylor & Francis Group.

Cameron ulcer/erosion: A mucosal disruption located within a hiatal hernia sac that can cause upper GI bleeding. Treatment may involve endoscopic hemostasis with clips or electrocautery, acid suppression therapy, or both.

***Campylobacter*-like organism (CLO) test:** A commercially available kit in which gastric biopsy samples are placed in a urea-containing medium to detect the presence of *H pylori* in the stomach. If *H pylori* is present, the urea is metabolized and ammonia is released. The kit is designed to detect elevated levels of ammonia to diagnose an *H pylori* infection. *Campylobacter*-like organism is the original name used to describe the bacteria now known as *H pylori.*

Candida: A group of fungal organisms that normally reside within the human oral cavity, skin, and female genitalia. They can become pathogenic, called candidiasis, when a patient's normal flora is disturbed, classically when an antibiotic is administered or when he or she is in an immunocompromised state. Common sites of candidiasis include the mouth, esophagus, bladder, and bloodstream.

candidal esophagitis: A condition when *Candida* proliferates and inflames the esophagus, leading to the endoscopic appearance of white plaques in the esophagus with associated esophageal inflammation. Odynophagia and dysphagia are commonly associated symptoms. Diagnosis is made by endoscopy, and first-line treatment is with oral or intravenous fluconazole. This disease can be an AIDS-defining illness or unrelated to AIDS but most often occurs in individuals who are immunosuppressed.

cannabinoid hyperemesis syndrome: A syndrome affecting chronic marijuana users that presents as cyclical episodes of nausea, vomiting, and abdominal pain often requiring hospitalization secondary to dehydration. Hot baths and showers can relieve the symptoms, and patients may bathe multiple times per day. Symptoms resolve when marijuana use ceases but resume if the patient restarts its use.

cannabinoid receptor: Found throughout the body, with the majority located in the brain. When activated, GI tract motility may decrease, appetite may increase, and pain response may be blunted; *also called* the tetrahydrocannabinol receptor.

cannulation: Successful entry of the bile duct or pancreatic duct during an ERCP. It can also refer to when a tube is inserted into the body for the purpose of delivering a substance, usually medication or fluid, or obtaining a sample.

capillary hemangioma: Benign tumors derived from capillaries, usually found on the skin of infants. They can also present on the skin of patients with chronic liver disease and are typically asymptomatic but may clue the clinician to the presence of chronic liver disease.

capsule endoscopy/enteroscopy: *See* wireless capsule endoscopy.

caput medusae: Dilated abdominal wall veins encircling the umbilicus in a serpentine fashion as a consequence of portal hypertension recanalizing the paraumbilical veins. This term makes reference to Medusa from Greek mythology, whose hair was turned into serpents.

carcinoid syndrome: A constellation of symptoms including flushing, diarrhea, right-sided heart failure, wheezing, and weight loss associated with the release of vasoactive substances, including serotonin, by metastatic carcinoid tumors. The diagnosis is made when high levels of serotonin and its metabolite 5-hydroxyindoleacetic acid are detected in the urine. Treatment involves providing symptomatic relief with agents such as bronchodilators, loperamide, histamine antagonists, and diuretics. Octreotide is also helpful in controlling symptoms.

carcinoid tumor: An abnormal proliferation of neuroendocrine tissue that can secrete a variety of hormones, including serotonin, gastrin, insulin, gastric inhibitory polypeptide, and vasoactive intestinal peptide (VIP). Common lesion sites include the appendix, ileum, rectum, bronchi, and liver, although they are typically metastatic if in the liver. When present in the liver, carcinoid syndrome can often occur.

carcinomatosis: Cancer that has spread throughout the body, particularly located on the omentum or mesentery. Cancers most often associated with carcinomatosis include ovarian, colon, pancreatic, and mesothelioma; *also called* carcinosis.

carcinosis: *Another term for* carcinomatosis.

cardia: The proximal stomach, located between the gastroesophageal junction and the gastric fundus. It is a common site for gastric varices to be located when present in patients with portal hypertension.

Caroli's disease: A congential cystic dilatation of the intrahepatic bile ducts that can lead to recurrent cholangitis, abscesses, and stone formation. Treatment includes ursodiol to decrease stone formation, antibiotics to treat or prevent cholangitis, and endoscopic and surgical management, as needed. This condition carries an increased risk of cholangiocarcinoma; *also called* Type V choledochal cyst; *see* Caroli's syndrome when associated with hepatic fibrosis.

Caroli's syndrome: Autosomal recessive inherited disorder of intrahepatic bile duct dilatation and associated hepatic fibrosis that can lead to portal hypertension and liver failure, often culminating in liver transplantation; *see* Caroli's disease.

catamenial: Synonymous with the menstrual cycle. Certain disease states are described as catamenial in nature if they coincide temporally with menses (eg, endometriosis pain).

caustic esophagitis: Damage to the esophagus secondary to accidental chemical ingestion, most often from an acid or alkali substance. A history of caustic esophagitis increases the future risk of squamous cell carcinoma of the esophagus more than 1000-fold.

cavernous hemangioma: Most common benign mass found in the liver composed of a tangling of blood vessels. Usually asymptomatic and does not require treatment. Large hemangiomas may press against the liver capsule and cause pain; resection may be indicated in this instance.

cecal volvulus: Twisting of the cecum around its mesentery that can compress local blood vessels, leading to ischemia or infarction. On abdominal radiography, it classically appears as a large kidney-shaped dilatation in the left upper quadrant. Decompression using a rectally introduced tube, colonoscopy, or surgery is often needed.

cecum: Most proximal portion of the colon, located between the terminal ileum and ascending colon. In addition, reaching this location during a colonoscopy is a quality measure of a complete examination. The appendix originates in the cecum.

celiac disease: An autoimmune disorder leading to a malabsorptive state in which the dietary component gluten triggers injury to intestinal villi. Treatment requires strict adherence to a gluten-free diet and lifestyle. The gold standard for diagnosis is intestinal biopsy. Serologic markers, including tissue transglutaminase and anti-endomysial antibody, are also characteristically positive; *also called* gluten-sensitive enteropathy; *see* Appendix 22.

ceruloplasmin: A protein that circulates in the blood that uniquely binds and transports copper. Decreased levels can be a sign of Wilson's disease. Also an acute phase reactant, levels of ceruloplasmin are influenced by infection or inflammation and can be increased in these situations.

Chagas disease: Infection with *Trypanosoma cruzi,* a parasite endemic to parts of Central and Latin America but can also be found in the southern United States. Humans are typically infected via an insect vector, the triatomine "kissing" bug. Approximately 20% to 30% of those with chronic infection may develop cardiac arrhythmias, congestive heart failure, and dilatation of the esophagus or colon. The esophageal appearance of megaesophagus may mimic achalasia. This infection can also be transmitted via blood transfusion or as a transplant-transmitted infection and, since 2005, is among the many infections screened for by the American Red Cross in donated blood.

Charcot's triad: The concomitant occurrence of three symptoms— fever, jaundice, and right upper quandrant pain—that are highly associated with acute cholangitis.

chemoembolization: A procedure performed by an interventional radiologist in which chemotherapeutic agents are injected directly into the blood supply feeding a tumor, after which the blood vessel is embolized to ensure the agent stays in the area of the tumor. Commonly used in the treatment of hepatocellular carcinoma. Different combinations of chemotherapeutic agents have been tried, and there is no one standard combination currently used.

chief cells: Cells found in the stomach that store and release pepsinogen, an enzyme involved in protein metabolism.

Chilaiditi syndrome: The presence of a loop of bowel in between the diaphragm and the liver. It is a possible cause of abdominal pain, but more commonly it is identified incidentally during abdominal imaging. It can be confused for a diaphragmatic injury or the presence of intraperitoneal air.

Child-Pugh-Turcotte classification: A risk stratification system used to characterize the severity of liver disease. It consists of classes A, B, and C and can be used to predict survival and complications related to surgery in patients with chronic liver disease. This classification was previously used to determine who could qualify for a liver transplant but has been replaced by the Model for End-Stage Liver Disease (MELD) score in the United States. Components of the scoring include serum albumin, total bilirubin, INR, severity of ascites, and severity of encephalopathy.

Chinese liver fluke: *Another term for* Clonorchis sinensis.

cholangiocarcinoma: Cancer of the bile ducts that can occur in ducts inside (intrahepatic) or outside (extrahepatic) the liver. Treatment is highly variable depending on the location and stage of disease at diagnosis. The diagnosis is often made by ERCP with brushings or cholangioscopy and biopsy. Surgical resection offers the best chance of long-term survival in early stage disease, and liver transplantation in combination with chemotherapy is sometimes an option for unresectable hilar lesions or cholangiocarcinoma arising in the background of primary sclerosing cholangitis.

cholangiogram: An imaging study of the biliary tree during which contrast dye is injected directly into the bile ducts percutaneously or during an ERCP or endoscopic ultrasound (EUS). This study is helpful in the diagnosis of biliary obstruction, stricture, choledocholithiasis, or malignancy. When completed during an ERCP, therapeutic intervention can be offered simultaneously.

cholangiopathy: A disease process that results in biliary ductal damage. Causes include infection, such as HIV/AIDS, ischemia, and autoimmune triggers.

cholangioscopy: Endoscopic evaluation of the bile or pancreatic ducts using a small camera fed through a standard duodenoscope's working channel. Cholangioscopy is a helpful procedure in the detection of cholangiocarcinoma, biliary strictures, intraductal papillary mucinous neoplasms, and complicated choledocholithiasis; *also known as* SpyGlass (Boston Scientific).

cholangitis: Inflammation of the bile ducts, usually secondary to a bacterial infection. Classically, it presents with Charcot's triad of fever, jaundice, and right upper quadrant pain. When it is severe, shock and altered mental status may also be present. Treatment requires antibiotics and decompression of the biliary tree.

cholatestasis: A pathologic change seen on liver biopsy characterized by cellular swelling from bile salt deposition, typically occurring in zone 1.

cholecystectomy: Surgical removal of the gallbladder, which can be performed using an open or laparoscopic procedure or via NOTES. It is commonly performed for gallstone-related disease, including biliary colic, acute cholecystitis, and chronic cholecystitis, and is one of the most commonly performed abdominal surgeries.

cholecystitis: Inflammation of the gallbladder wall often associated with a gram-negative bacterial infection following obstruction of the cystic duct with a gallstone. It can also occur in the absence of stone disease, in which case it is referred to as acalculous. Diagnosis is typically made by ultrasound, although a HIDA scan, CT, or MRI can also be diagnostic. Antibiotics and cholecystectomy are usually used for treatment.

cholecystoduodenal fistula: An abnormal connection that forms between the gallbladder and the duodenum, usually as a result of a large gallstone. It is commonly associated with gallstone ileus because a large stone passing through the fistula can become stuck at the ileocecal valve, leading to a functional bowel obstruction.

cholecystokinin: A hormone released by cells in the intestines when encountering amino acids, peptides, and fatty acids that induces a multitude of physiologic phenomena in the GI tract. Primarily, it stimulates enzymatic secretion from the pancreas, contracts the gallbladder, and relaxes the sphincter of Oddi. It also enhances the effect of secretin, augmenting bicarbonate secretion from the pancreas. These processes all aid in the digestion of fat and protein present in the GI tract.

cholecystostomy: Drainage tube placement into a distended gallbladder through the skin that is performed as an alternative to cholecystectomy in patients who are at high surgical risk.

choledochal cyst: A congenital bile duct cystic anomaly that is further categorized into 5 types based on location using the Todani classification system. Type I is the most common (80% to 90%) and is a sac-like dilatation of the common bile duct. Type II is a common bile duct diverticulum. Type III is called a choledochocele. Type IV involves multiple cystic dilatations of the intrahepatic or extrahepatic bile ducts. Type V is called Caroli's disease. Choledochal cysts occur more commonly in women and people of Asian descent and carry an increased liftetime risk of cholangiocarcinoma. Surgical treatment is the only curative therapy for all types, although ERCP and sphincterotomy may help prevent cholangitis for smaller, type III choledochal cysts.

choledochocele: A type III choledochal cyst characterized by dilatation of only the intraduodenal segment of the common bile duct. Choledochoceles smaller than 3 cm can be treated with endoscopic sphincterotomy, whereas larger ones are resected; *see* choledochal cyst.

choledocholithiasis: The presence of gallstones in the common bile duct or a branch of the biliary tree. Although stones in the gallbladder can be left alone, stones in the biliary tree are generally removed because they often cause pain, elevated liver tests, and jaundice and can predispose individuals to cholangitis and liver abscess formation. The diagnosis can be made using an abdominal ultrasound, CT scan, magnetic resonance cholangio-pancreatography, or ERCP. An ERCP is the preferred method for stone removal. When ERCP is unsuccessful, surgical bile duct exploration is indicated.

cholelithiasis: The presence of gallstones in the gallbladder. This term only implies that stones exist and does not imply symptoms. Instead, the term *biliary colic* is used to describe postprandial abdominal pain or dyspepsia associated with the presence of stones; *see* biliary colic; *see* Appendix 26.

cholestasis: A disruption in the usual bile flow pattern from the liver parenchyma to the duodenum by either mechanical obstruction of the biliary tree or a hepatocelluar process, such as infection, inflammation, metabolic causes, or drug injury, that causes impaired secretion of bile by the liver cells. Symptoms may include jaundice and pruritus.

chromoendoscopy: A procedure in which a dye is sprayed onto the mucosa of the GI tract in an attempt to enhance detection of abnormal tissue. Potential applications include evaluation for Barrett's esophagus and for adenomatous polyps in the colon. This technique is not widely used due to the additional time needed for the procedure, the lack of definitive value compared with white light (regular) endoscopy, and a relative paucity of trained clinicians familiar with the technique.

chronic calcific pancreatitis: The presence of calcium deposits in the pancreas on imaging, typically CT scan, in patients with chronic pancreatitis. This is associated most often with alcohol-related chronic pancreatitis. Incidental finding of pancreatic calcifications on cross-sectional imaging should prompt an evaluation for chronic pancreatitis.

chronic cholecystitis: Long-term inflammation of the gallbladder wall almost exclusively due to the presence of cholelithiasis. It may be asymptomatic for years before presenting with biliary colic, acute cholecystitis, or more severe complications, including abscess or perforation. Symptoms may include postprandial right upper quadrant abdominal pain or nausea. A cholecystectomy is performed as treatment.

chronic constipation: Long-term difficulty with moving bowels lasting more than 6 months; *also called* functional constipation. Patients must meet specific criteria (Rome criteria) to be diagnosed with this condition, including at least 2 of the following symptoms: fewer than 3 bowel movements per week; 25% or more of the defecations are associated with straining, lumpy or hard stools; sensation of incomplete evacuation; sensation of anorectal obstruction or blockage; or the need for manual maneuvers to defecate. Abdominal pain is not usually a major symptom and, if present, a diagnosis of IBD is usually more appropriate. Treatment includes laxatives, fiber supplementation, stool softeners, and dietary/lifestyle modification.

chronic gastritis: Inflammation of the stomach over a long period of time leading to destruction of gastric glands, often presenting with abdominal pain or dyspepsia. Causes include drug injury (NSAIDs use), alcohol, autoimmune-related inflammation, and *H pylori* infection. Endoscopy with gastric mucosal biopsies is the diagnostic procedure of choice. Treatment typically involves elimination of the inciting etiology and acid suppressive therapy.

chronic intestinal pseudo-obstruction: A motility disorder of the GI tract in which patients present with chronic symptoms mimicking bowel obstruction (eg, nausea, vomiting, abdominal pain, decreased flatus, air-fluid levels on radiography, and constipation) without an obvious obstruction. Treatment is focused on symptom management. This condition can predispose individuals to small intestinal bacterial overgrowth.

chronic pancreatitis: Long-standing and persistent inflammation of the pancreas as a result of toxic (alcohol), autoimmune, mechanical obstruction (stones/strictures), genetic, metabolic, or idiopathic causes leading to irreversible changes in the pancreas. This results in exocrine or endocrine dysfunction that can present with malabsorption, abdominal pain, nausea, vomiting, or diabetes mellitus. Treatment is mostly palliative and includes oral pancreatic enzymes supplementation, endoscopic stone extraction and stenting, and blood glucose control.

cirrhosis: Advanced fibrosis of the liver as a result of chronic inflammation caused by viral, autoimmune, toxic, or metabolic injury. The fibrosis leads to anatomic changes in the liver, including coarsened surface, nodularity, medial segment atrophy, and caudate lobe hypertrophy and results in the development of portal hypertension. It can be compensated or decompensated (associated with ascites, variceal bleeding, portosystemic encephalopathy, hepatic hydrothorax, hepatopulmonary syndrome, hepatorenal syndrome, or liver cancer). When cirrhosis is decompensated, liver transplant may be life-sustaining; *also called* end-stage liver disease.

clean-based ulcer: A lower risk type of GI ulceration characterized by the absence of active bleeding or stigmata of recent bleeding on endoscopy. The risk of rebleeding is less than 10% when this type of ulcer is diagnosed, and outpatient management with proton pump inhibitor medications can usually be safely pursued.

Clonorchis sinensis: A parasitic worm indigenous to China, Vietnam, and Korea. Humans become infected when they eat undercooked fish previously infected with *C sinensis*. After ingestion, the worm can grow within the bile ducts, causing biliary obstruction, cholangitis, or both. It increases the lifetime risk for developing cholangiocarcinoma; *also called* the Chinese liver fluke.

C-loop: Describes the first three parts of the duodenum due to its c-shaped curvature in the abdomen.

Clostridium difficile: A gram-positive, spore-forming, toxin-producing bacterium that is the leading cause of hospital-acquired diarrhea. Spores are ingested and proliferate in patients who are taking antibiotics or who are immunocompromised. Diarrhea can be severe, and dehydration is not uncommon. Stool assays are used for diagnosis and can detect antigen, toxin, culture, or DNA. Hand washing with soap and water can help prevent spread because it is not killed by standard alcohol-based hand rubs. Severe infection can cause toxic megacolon. Antibiotics, including metronidazole, oral vancomycin, or fidaxomicin, are typically used for treatment.

clubbing: A physical examination finding in which the curvature of the fingernail is lost due to an increase in spongy connective tissue below it. It is associated with cardiopulmonary disease and cirrhosis.

CMV colitis: *See* cytomegalovirus colitis.

CMV esophagitis: *See* cytomegalovirus esophagitis.

cobalamin: *See* vitamin B_{12}.

coffee ground emesis: A dark, granular type of emesis that resembles coffee grounds. It is characteristic of upper GI bleeding. The differential diagnosis includes peptic ulcer disease, gastritis, esophagitis, duodenitis, malignancy, Dieulafoy's lesion, portal hypertensive gastropathy, or less likely variceal hemorrhage. Acid suppressive therapy and upper endocsopy are usually the next steps in the evaluation and treatment.

cold biopsy: Removal of a piece of tissue with biopsy forceps during an endoscopy, without the assistance of electrocautery. This is the standard endoscopic biopsy. Polyps can also be removed using this technique if they are small.

colectomy: The surgical excision of all or part of the colon. If the entire colon is removed, the term *total colectomy* is more accurate. A partial colectomy refers to a segmental resection. Indications include CRC, dysplastic ulcerative colitis, complicated diverticular disease, and obstruction.

collagenous colitis: A type of microscopic colonic inflammation (microscopic colitis) presenting as watery diarrhea and often affecting the elderly or patients with autoimmune conditions, such as celiac disease, but having a characteristically normal endoscopic appearance. Biopsies demonstrate a chronic inflammatory infiltrate in the mucosa with a collagen band in the lamina propria. Treatment options include budesonide, mesalamine, steroids, and bismuth.

colitis: Inflammation of the large intestine with many possible causes, including IBD, infection, ischemia, and drug-induced injury. Symptoms include abdominal pain, diarrhea with or without blood, fevers, and fecal urgency. The diagnostic workup includes a careful history, stool studies, imaging, and often colonoscopy with biopsies. Treatment is targeted to the etiology.

colon cancer: One of the most common cancers in the United States and worldwide. It may be completely asymptomatic at diagnosis or be suspected in patients with abdominal pain, change in bowel habits, weight loss, or bleeding. Colon cancer typically refers to adenocarcionma of the colon, and most adenocarcinomas arise from an existing type of polyp called an adenoma. A screening colonoscopy can remove adenomatous polyps before they become cancer. Treatment depends on the stage at diagnosis. If confined to the colon, surgery can be curative. If it has advanced beyond the colon, adjuvant treatment with chemotherapy with or without radiation is usually indicated.

colonic: Of or pertaining to the colon. Also, an infusion of water or other substances into the colon with reported benefits of cleansing toxins and preventing or treating constipation. Little scientific data support the use of colonics for medical purposes, although they are popular and can be administered by non-healthcare professionals.

colonic inertia: *See* slow transit constipation.

colonic ischemia: Low blood flow to a portion of the colon leading to (usually) reversible damage of the colon. Patients may present with abdominal pain and lower GI bleeding (hematochezia), usually occurring after some type of stressor, such as prolonged fasting, severe dehydration, abdominal surgery, or repair of an aortic aneurysm. Treatment is aimed at improving colonic perfusion with intravenous fluids and antibiotics if infection is present or suspected. Severe cases can cause colonic perforation and require urgent surgery.

colonic perforation: A tear in the lining of the colon that can occur iatrogenically (eg, during a colonoscopy) or pathologically (eg, Crohn's disease or malignancy related). It can occur intraperitoneally or retroperitoneally. Intraperitoneal perforation requires urgent surgical intervention. Retroperitoneal perforations may be amenable to endoscopic closure or conservative measures, such as bowel rest and antibiotics. There is a high morbidity and mortality associated with colonic perforation due to stool spilling out into the peritoneal cavity and putting the patient at risk of sepsis.

colonic stent: A device usually made of a metallic mesh inserted into the colon to relieve a stricture. It is usually placed via colonoscopy but can also be placed under fluoroscopy by interventional radiology. It is most often used to relieve large bowel A obstruction caused by a malignant colonic stricture either as a bridge to surgery, or as destination therapy. Successful placement may decrease the need for a stoma creation. A major risk of placement is colonic perforation.

colonic stricture: A narrowing of the colonic lumen that can lead to symptoms of bowel obstruction, including constipation, nausea, vomiting, and abdominal pain. It can be benign (Crohn's disease, diverticular-associated, ischemic-associated) or malignant (colon cancer). Radiographs, CT scans, barium enemas, or a colonoscopy can aide in making the diagnosis. Treatment depends on the etiology of the stricture but includes endoscopic dilatation, surgical diversion, surgical excision, or medical therapy.

colonic transit test: A radiologic test used in the diagnosis of colonic inertia. The patient ingests several small radio-opaque markers, called Sitz markers, and radiographs are taken at specific time intervals after ingestion. The location of markers at each time point is used to measure the colonic transit. This test requires several days to complete.

colonic ulcer: Erosions of the large intestinal mucosa that put patients at risk for a lower GI bleeding, abdominal pain, and diarrhea. They can occur as a result of chronic inflammatory conditions, such as IBD or Behçet's disease, or can form acutely from ischemia or infection. Colon cancers can also ulcerate the mucosa, so malignancy is also in the differential diagnosis.

colonic varices: Dilated, swollen venous structures located in the colon that form as a result of portal hypertension. The colon is a rare site for variceal formation in patients with portal hypertension, occurring less than 5% of the time. Patients present with bright red blood per rectum or darker lower GI bleeding. Most incidences will spontaneously stop, although massive bleeding can occur and presents a significant risk of morbidity and mortality. Efforts to correct portal hypertension with transjugular intrahepatic portosystemic shunt (TIPS) or liver transplantation may be indicated for recurrent or refractory bleeding.

colonoscopy: An endoscopic procedure in which a long, flexible tube with a light and video camera at the end is inserted through the anus and advanced proximally in the colon to the cecum and ileocecal valve. It is performed for several indications, most commonly for colon cancer screening, polyp removal, diagnosis of chronic diarrhea, and evaluation of GI bleeding. Biopsy specimens can be obtained through the scope, if indicated. Colonoscopy is considered the gold standard for colonic polyp and cancer detection. It is usually performed with sedation and requires a purgative bowel preparation to allow adequate mucosal visualization.

common bile duct: The distal segment of the biliary tree that forms from the confluence of the common hepatic duct and cystic duct that drains through the ampulla of Vater into the second portion of the duodenum. All of the bile made in the liver eventually reaches the common bile duct before being used in digestion.

common bile duct obstruction: Blockage of the major drainage system of the liver before it enters the duodenum, leading to jaundice, elevated liver tests, right upper quadrant abdominal pain, nausea, and risk for cholangitis. Common etiologies for obstruction include choledocholithiasis, stricture, and external compression from malignancy of the pancreas. Treatment usually involves biliary decompression by ERCP, surgery, or percutaneous drain placement.

common bile duct stricture: Narrowing of the common bile duct by either a benign or malignant process that can cause cholangitis, abdominal pain, jaundice, and difficulty eating fatty foods. Treatment is the same as those listed for other causes of bile duct obstruction.

complementary and alternative medicine: The use of therapy that does not fall under the umbrella of conventional medicine as practiced by allopathic and osteopathic physicians. This can include mind–body techniques (such as yoga and meditation), massage, and supplements, including herbal remedies and probiotics.

computed tomography (CT): An imaging modality that uses radiography technology to capture multiple, thinly sliced radiographs taken over a short period of time to aid in the diagnosis and management of many conditions. CT can be performed over any area of the body and is commonly used in gastroenterology in the evaluation of abdominal pain, IBD, and liver masses. Additions of contrast agents orally, intravenously, or both enhance the diagnostic yield of the test.

confidence interval: A statistic that is used to demonstrate a range of values in which the factor being studied has a predetermined probability to fall between. For example, a 95% confidence interval of 2 to 5 indicates a 95% probability that the outcome measured is truly between 2 and 5. If a value falls within the confidence interval, it is unlikely to have occurred by chance (1-confidence interval).

confluent hepatic necrosis: A pathologic finding on a liver biopsy of a patient with acute hepatitis, often due to drug injury, such as acetaminophen, or fulminant autoimmune hepatitis. The more necrosis seen on biopsy, the more unlikely the patient's liver is to recover, often necessitating a liver transplantation. On imaging, the liver may appear cirrhotic but in actuality the liver is collapsing on itself due to cellular death; this can occur in an irregular manner, mimicking a nodular appearance on ultrasound or cross-sectional imaging.

Congo Red stain: A dye used on histologic specimens to diagnose amyloidosis. The stain makes amyloid deposits appear pink or red under light microscopy and greenish under polarized microscopy. This greenish hue is referred to as "apple-green birefringence."

constipation: A change in the number or quality of bowel movements that is manifested by decreased frequency (less than 3 times per week) or harder, lumpier stools that are difficult to pass, often requiring straining or manual maneuvers. It can come on acutely (eg, in a patient prescribed an opiate analgesic) or be chronic (*see also* chronic constipation). Treatment is aimed at reducing precipitating triggers, and relief can usually be obtained with stool softeners, laxatives, fiber supplementation, and dietary/lifestyle modification.

copper: A mineral that is required as a cofactor for multiple enzymatic processes in the body. It is found in shellfish, nuts, and legumes. Deficiency can lead to anemia, osteopenia, neurologic changes, and delayed growth. Excess copper, known as Wilson's disease, can cause cirrhosis, liver failure, neurologic changes, and hemolytic anemia.

core-needle biopsy: Placement of a hollow-bore needle into the target organ to obtain a thin piece of tissue. It is used to obtain a sample that includes the native architecture; *compare* fine-needle aspiration, which aims to remove abnormal cells only. This is the most common method of performing a liver biopsy.

councilman bodies: A pathological finding in the liver associated with yellow fever caused by eosinophilic degeneration of the hepatocytes, which is associated with condensed nuclear chromatin. This pathology is not usually determined while a patient is infected with yellow fever because biopsies are not recommended due to hemorrhagic risks and has been mostly characterized on postmortem examinations.

Cowden's syndrome: An autosomal dominant inherited condition associated with PTEN mutations, a type of PHTS. Patients develop multiple hamartomatous polyps in the GI tract, as well as skin lesions (including trichilemmomas and verrucous papules) and macrocephaly. This syndrome carries an increased lifetime risk of breast, kidney, thyroid, endometrial, and colorectal cancers.

Crail's syndrome: An inherited condition in which patients develop hundreds of polyps in their GI tract in addition to central nervous system malignancies. It is thought to be a variant of FAP and is caused by a mutation in a DNA mismatch repair gene; *also called* Turcot's syndrome.

Crigler-Najjar syndrome: A rare inherited condition of impaired bilirubin conjugation that puts patients at risk for kernicterus and brain injury. Type 1 affects neonates and treatment with bilirubin lights is imperative, although many patients require liver transplantation. Type 2 affects patients later in childhood and is more indolent, but kernicterus can still occur and life expectancy without transplant is less than 30 years.

Crohn's disease: A type of IBD that can involve any part of the GI tract, from the mouth to the anus. The most common site of inflammation is the terminal ileum and the inflammation is transmural. Patients present with fever, watery or bloody diarrhea (or both), and abdominal pain. GI complications include fistulas, strictures, and bowel obstruction. Extra-intestinal manifestations may include arthritis, uveitis, iritis, and dermatologic conditions, including pyoderma gangrenosum and erythema nodosum. Diagnosis is made clinically using data obtained from labs, imaging, endoscopy, and biopsy. There are several medications used for Crohn's disease, including 5-aminosalicylic acid drugs, steroids, antibiotics, immunomodulators, and biologic drugs. Surgery is necessary in more than one-third of patients with Crohn's disease to control symptoms or treat complications; *also called* regional enteritis.

Crohn's disease activity index (CDAI): A research tool used to help quantify how well certain medications treat Crohn's disease. The index includes input from the following variables: the average number of patient-reported stools per day, average abdominal pain rating (none to severe), general well-being (well to terrible), complications of Crohn's disease (joint, eye, skin, fistulas, perianal disease, fevers), presence of an abdominal mass, degree of anemia, and weight changes. Each value is assigned a specific number of points, with lower total points suggesting less symptomatic disease. A score less than 150 usually indicates that the patient is in clinical remission. It is not routinely used in clinical practice but allows for an objective measure of symptoms during a research study.

Cronkhite-Canada syndrome: A rare, noninherited disease characterized by cutaneous and GI involvement. The GI involvement presents as multiple hamartomatous polyps throughout the GI tract that can cause significant bleeding and protein-losing enteropathy or diarrhea. The syndrome is also characterized by alopecia, skin hyperpigmentation, and onychodystrophy (the loss of finger and toe nails). It carries a mortality rate of more than 50% at 5 years, and death often occurs as a result of bleeding, heart failure, or sepsis.

Cruveilhier-Baumgarten's sign: The presence of an abdominal bruit over the umbilical or paraumbilical veins. In an adult patient with portal hypertension, it signifies the presence of a recanalized portal vein.

cryoablation: Destruction of tissue using extreme cold to induce local ischemic injury and cell apotosis. When applied through a catheter, it can be used endoscopically in the treatment of dysplastic Barrett's esophagus or percutaneously in the treatment of hepatic neoplasms.

cryoglobulinemia: A type of small vessel vasculitis caused by deposition of immune complexes into the small vessels that is often triggered by viral hepatitis, including hepatitis B and C. Symptoms include purpuric or petechial rashes (particularly of the distal lower extremities), peripheral neuropathy, renal failure, and, rarely, other organ involvement. In hepatitis-associated cryoglobulinemia, treatment of the hepatitis improves the cryoglobulinemia. In more severe presentations, corticosteroids, plasma exchange, rituximab, or cyclophosphamide may be necessary.

crypt abscess: A classic histological finding of the colonic mucosa in patients with active IBD, particularly ulcerative colitis, in which white blood cells are attracted to the colonic crypts.

cryptitis: A histological finding associated with IBD, but one that occurs earlier than crypt abscesses. Neutrophils invade the intestinal crypts, causing inflammation. Over time, this cryptitis can lead to crypt abscess formation.

cryptogenic cirrhosis: End-stage liver disease of an unknown etiology. Many historical cases of this disease likely resulted from nonalcoholic steatohepatitis or surreptitious alcohol-related injury.

curcumin: Found in the Indian spice turmeric, a supplement or herbal substance that has been used primarily in Ayurvedic medicine but has gained popularity in Western medicine. Common conditions for which it has been studied include for pain relief in osteoarthritis, Alzheimer's disease, atherosclerosis, diabetes mellitus, liver inflammation, and colon and pancreatic cancer.

cyclic vomiting syndrome: A clinical syndrome characterized by episodes of severe nausea and vomiting that can last hours or days, followed by periods in which patients are completely asymptomatic. The symptomatic episodes are usually triggered by an illness, including the common cold. This condition has been linked to migraines, and medications used for migraines, such as triptans, may be beneficial. In addition, ondansetron can be used for symptomatic relief. Fluids should be provided to avoid dehydration.

cyclophilin inhibitor: A new class of medication being investigated for the treatment of hepatitis C virus (HCV). May be one of many potential targets to help enable interferon-free treatment for HCV. The first molecule in this class is called alisporivir.

cystadenoma: A benign neoplasm with malignant potential that can occur in many organs, including the pancreas, liver, appendix, and ovaries. Of these locations, the pancreas is the most common GI site for cystadenomas. Pancreatic cystadenomas can be serous or mucinous and are often discovered incidentally when a patient undergoes abdominal imaging for another reason. Alternatively, patients may present with pain, acute pancreatitis, nausea, or vomiting. EUS with fine-needle aspiration can help determine the malignant potential and guide treatment, which can include observation or surgical resection.

cystic fibrosis: An autosomal recessive disorder most often seen in White patients that is characterized by recurrent sinusitis, frequent pneumonia, and bronchiectasis that ultimately leads to respiratory failure. Pancreatic insufficiency is also characteristically common, leading to steatorrhea and severe weight loss. The diagnosis is made using sweat chloride testing or genetic screening. A pulmonologist is usually involved in the management of these patients but, from a GI perspective, most patients require pancreatic enzyme replacement.

cystic pancreatic lesion: Fluid-filled collections or growths found in the pancreas that can be due to several causes. The most common lesion is a pseudocyst, although other types of cystic lesions include serous cystadenoma, mucinous cystic neoplasm, intraductal papillary mucinous neoplasm, solid pseudopapillary neoplasm, or, less likely, pancreatic adenocarcinoma. Cystic lesions can also be seen in genetic disorders, such as von Hippel-Lindau disease and autosomal dominant polycystic kidney disease. Diagnostic tests include CT scan, MRI, and EUS with or without fine-needle aspiration. Treatment depends on whether symptoms exist and whether the lesion has a high risk of malignant transformation.

cytochrome: One of a group of proteins located in the mitochondria involved in the generation of energy for the cell using electron transport to create adenosine triphosphate. Some cytochromes are also involved in the metabolism, oxidation, and reduction of many processes in the body.

cytochrome P450: A specific type of cytochrome that is important in drug metabolism. People can have genetic variations of enzyme types in this class that can lead to variable responses to medication. In addition, cytochrome P450 enzymes can be inhibited or induced by medications, alcohol, and certain foods that can put patients at risk for toxicity or less than desired efficacy of prescribed medications.

cytokine: A small protein molecule that acts as a signal from one cell to another. Cytokines are created in one cell and can affect that same cell (eg, IL-2 in helper T-cells) or another cell (eg, interferon-gamma).

***Cytomegalovirus* (CMV):** A DNA virus in the herpesvirus family that can cause a wide array of diseases affecting multiple organ systems. In healthy individuals, CMV can cause a mononucleosis-like syndrome but is generally asymptomatic. In patients who are immunocompromised, the virus can infect almost every organ, including the esophagus, liver, small intestine, colon, lungs, and retina. CMV is also a "torch" infection (ie, if contracted by a fetus in utero, it can cause a well-characterized congenital infection in neonates leading to jaundice, rash, premature birth, brain calcifications, mental retardation, and hepatosplenomegaly).

cytomegalovirus colitis: A severe infection of the colon seen primarily in patients who are immunocompromised, especially in patients with AIDS, leading to the formation of ulcers and inflammation. In addition, is it commonly seen in patients with IBD because the virus seems to demonstrate a tropism toward the inflamed tissue. Diagnosis requires biopsy with immunohistochemical analysis or a tissue culture. Intravenous ganciclovir is typically the initial treatment.

cytomegalovirus enteritis: An infection of the small bowel usually seen in patients with AIDS or those who are otherwise immunocompromised. Diagnosis requires biopsy with immunohistochemical analysis or tissue culture. Initial treatment is typically with intravenous ganciclovir.

cytomegalovirus esophagitis: An infection of the esophagus primarily seen in patients who are immunocompromised, especially those with AIDS. Pathognomonic shallow ulcers can be found throughout the esophagus, but ulceration is not mandatory for the diagnosis. Biopsy with immunohistochemistry or a tissue culture is diagnostic. Biopsies should be taken from the center or base of the ulcerations for the highest yield. Initial treatment is typically with intravenous gangiclovir.

cytomegalovirus hepatitis: A form of CMV infection leading to inflammation in the liver. It can occur in patients who are immunocompetent or immunocompromised. There is a risk factor for organ rejection if it occurs in an allograft liver.

D-xylose absorption test: A test used to evaluate for small intestinal malabsorption. D-xylose is a type of sugar than can be absorbed by active transport and passive diffusion in the small intestine. To perform the test, after an overnight fast, the patient swallows 25 g of D-xylose, has a blood draw 1 hour later, and has his or her urine output collected for 5 hours. Concentrations of D-xylose are measured in the two samples. Low levels suggest an intestinal mucosal disease, such as celiac disease. Pancreatic insufficiency does not reduce the absorption of D-xylose, and the test would yield normal concentrations. False positive tests may occur in patients with ascites, bacterial overgrowth, or gastroparesis.

decompressing gastrostomy: Placement of a percutaneous endoscopic gastrostomy (PEG) tube, or surgically placed PEG tube, for decompression of a distended stomach as a result of a malignant or nonmalignant obstruction. A feeding jejunostomy is usually placed distal to the gastrostomy tube, and patients can simply open the gastrostomy to the air for venting if they feel nauseous or have abdominal bloating.

defecography: *See* barium defecography.

delta cell (D cell): Cells found in the gastric antrum and intestine that function primarily to produce somatostatin, an inhibitor of gastric acid section. In patients with *H pylori* infection of the gastric antrum, the gastritis causes injury to the D cells, inhibiting somatostatin release and leading to increased levels of serum gastrin.

descending colon: The section of colon located between the splenic flexure and the sigmoid. It is approximately 30 cm in length for most people. Its major physiologic role is that of a storage reservoir for feces before it is excreted, but it also helps in water absorption.

device-assisted enteroscopy: A burgeoning category of endoscopy that includes single and double balloon enteroscopy and spiral overtube-assisted enteroscopy for the diagnosis and management of small bowel lesions, including obscure GI bleeding. The use of devices to aid in propulsion of the scope allows for deeper depth of insertion and examination, with the potential to treat or diagnose more lesions without the need for abdominal surgical exploration.

diaphragmatic hernia: A protrusion of a portion of the stomach through a defect in the diaphragm, usually the esophageal hiatus, due to congenital weakness, incomplete fusion, or a posttraumatic rupture of the diaphragm. The most common site in adults is herniation through the esophageal hiatus. In newborns with congenital diaphragmatic hernias, the most common location is on the left side, posterolaterally. Congenital diaphragmatic hernias are associated with significant pulmonary complications, including pulmonary hypoplasia and pulmonary hypertension; surgical repair within a few days of birth is necessary for survival.

diaphragm disease: A lesion of the small intestine characteristically caused by the use of NSAIDs. The lesions are thin strictures of the intestine with diaphragm-like openings and are thought to be created by scar formation from ulcerations caused by NSAID use. This condition may cause intestinal obstruction and require surgical intervention if complete obstruction is present.

diarrhea: Loose stools that are objectively defined as more than 200 g of stool per day or more than three loose bowel movements in 1 day. It can be acute or chronic in duration and has a multitude of causes, not limited to infection, inflammation, medication-induced, or malabsorption. Treatment is generally supportive, but treatment targeted at the underlying condition or trigger is also appropriate and may include bulking agents, such as fiber, or medications that slow gut motility, such as loperamide.

diathermy coagulation: A method used to stop bleeding in the GI tract or as a result of surgery using cautery via a heated electrical current either flowing from one electrode to a fixed electrode (monopolar) or between 2 electrodes mounted in the same device (bipolar). Monopolar diathermy is a common way of cauterizing a bleeding ulcer found during endoscopy in the GI tract. Bipolar diathermy is more commonly used in the operating room.

diet: The summation of nutritional intake a person consumes. People may be instructed to follow specific diets based on disease status (eg, gluten-free diet for celiac disease or low-residue diet for active Crohn's disease). It can also be used as a verb, meaning to purposefully consume certain types of nutritional intake either for medical reasons or to lose weight by one's own volition. Dieticians are trained experts in the ordered administration of nutritional intake.

Dieulafoy's lesion: An abnormally large submucosal artery usually found in the proximal stomach but can also be located anywhere in the GI tract that is a rare cause of GI hemorrhage. It is often missed on initial endoscopy because it can bleed quickly and then spontaneously stop. It usually presents as hematemesis or melena and can be intermittent in nature. Once located endoscopically, a mechanical clip can be used to achieve hemostasis.

digital rectal examination: *See* rectal examination.

direct-acting antiviral agents (DAAs): Medications that directly inhibit enzymes within the HCV lifecycle, leading to increased rates of virologic response. The first-in-class DAAs were the protease inhibitors boceprevir and telaprevir. Prior to their development, hepatitis C treatment was nonspecific with interferon and ribavirin-based regimens, which promoted host immune responses to aid in viral eradication.

discriminant function (DF): A mathematical formula designed by American hepatologist Dr. Willis Maddrey to help estimate the severity of alcoholic hepatitis and to determine which patients with alcoholic hepatitis would most benefit from treatment with corticosteroids. A score > 32 predicts a severe course and corticosteroid therapy is advised if safe. DF = 4.6 × [prothrombin time (seconds) − control prothrombin time (seconds)] + serum bilirubin (mg/dL); *see* Appendix 5.

distal esophagus: The lower one-third of the esophagus. This area is often the site of inflammation (*called* esophagitis) caused by acid reflux exposure. It ends at the gastroesophageal junction, *also known as* the z-line.

diuresis: The act of removing excess fluid from the body using either intravenous or oral medication. Several targets exist for diuretic medications, including sodium reabsorption in the kidney's loop of Henle and aldosterone antagonism. Conditions associated with a proclivity for fluid overload, such as cirrhosis, congestive heart failure, and nephrotic syndrome, are the most common conditions in which diuresis is necessary.

diuretic: A medication used for diuresis; *see* diuresis.

diversion colitis: Inflammation of a segment of colon or rectum that is no longer in continuity with the GI tract, such as one that occurs after a diverting ileostomy or colostomy. It is thought to occur as a result of a deficiency in short chain fatty acids (SCFA) that provide nutrients to the colon. SCFA are usually created via bacterial metabolism of the fecal stream, which is absent in this anatomic alteration. Treatment is to reverse the diversion and restore the fecal stream. If that is not possible, SCFA enemas are effective for many patients.

diverticular abscess: A complication of acute diverticulitis in which a collection of pus forms adjacent to an area of diverticulitis. Clinically, it presents as worsening abdominal pain and fever or persistently elevated white blood cell count despite 2 to 3 days of treatment with antibiotics. A CT scan is the best method to diagnose the condition, and percutaneous drainage or surgery may be necessary.

diverticular-associated colitis: Inflammation of a segment of colon in the same vicinity as colonic diverticulosis. The diagnosis is difficult to distinguish from IBD, but generally it is more limited in extent and has a more benign course.

diverticulitis: Acute inflammation of a diverticulum, most often in the colon, presenting as abdominal pain, fever, and a change in bowel habits. Because diverticulosis is most common in the left colon, left lower quadrant pain is the most frequent location of pain. Right-sided diverticulitis may mimic appendicitis. Treatment includes antibiotics, bowel rest, and surgery in advanced or recurrent cases.

diverticulosis: The condition of having small pouch-like openings called diverticula in the GI tract. Most often, this condition is detected incidentally during a colonoscopy or CT scan, and most patients are asymptomatic. Less than one quarter of patients will have symptoms related to diverticulosis, including painless lower GI bleeding, abdominal pain, or acute inflammation (known as diverticulitis). It is a common finding in adults older than 50 years and is most commonly located in the sigmoid and descending colon.

Dor fundoplication: A surgical treatment for GERD most often used as part of the surgical management for achalasia in combination with a myotomy. The procedure reinforces the lower esophageal sphincter with a single flap placed 180 degrees anteriorly (instead of 360 degrees) to reduce the risk of obstruction in cases of poor esophageal motility; *also known as* a partial anterior fundoplication.

double balloon enteroscopy: A type of device-assisted enteroscopy used primarily to diagnose and treat small bowel abnormalities, particularly in patients with obscure GI bleeding. The procedure involves using a long flexible endoscope with a balloon built into the tip of the scope and passed through an overtube that also has a balloon on the tip. Insufflating and deflating the balloons in combination with specific pull-back techniques significantly decrease looping of the scope, and deep intubation of the small bowel is possible. It can be performed antegrade or retrograde. This technique can also be used for pancreaticobiliary procedures in patients with altered anatomy after gastric bypass or other biliary diversion procedures.

double bubble sign: A classic radiographic finding of duodenal obstruction in newborns seen on anteroposterior abdominal radiographs. It is diagnostic of duodenal obstruction, either by duodenal stenosis or atresia.

drug-drug interaction: When 2 or more drugs that are taken simultaneously affect the function of one or both of the drugs. An interaction may occur in the liver during drug metabolism or in the intestine during absorption. The effect may lead to drug toxicity if a drug level is increased or ineffectiveness if a level is decreased. Understanding how specific drugs are absorbed and metabolized in the body and choosing drugs unlikely to interact with one another can decrease the likelihood of significant interactions.

drug-induced colitis: A noninfectious cause of colonic mucosal inflammation that presents as bloody diarrhea, weight loss, and dehydration. NSAIDs, antibiotics, and certain stimulant laxatives are the most common drugs associated with colitis.

drug-induced liver injury: Liver test abnormalities and hepatocellular dysfunction that occur as a result of predictable or idiosyncratic drug injury. For example, acetaminophen follows a predictable rate of liver injury based on dose exposure, whereas many other medications or drugs may not. The clinical presentation and laboratory findings are highly variable. Treatment is aimed at cessation of the offending agent and supportive care. Liver transplantation may be required in severe cases associated with acute liver failure.

Drug Rash with Eosinophilia and Systemic Symptoms (DRESS): Observed 1 to 6 weeks after exposure to a drug. The classic association is with anticonvulsants but can occur from many medications including telaprevir, an HCV protease inhibitor. Classic symptoms include fever, maculopapular rash, facial swelling, lymphadenopathy, and liver test abnormalities. Cessation of the offending drug is paramount in management, along with supportive care.

dual energy x-ray absorptiometry (DEXA) scan: Imaging method used to measure bone mineral density. Results are reported as either T- or Z-scores. T-scores represent a comparison of the individual's results to the peak bone density of a younger population of the same race and gender. Z-scores compare individuals to an age-, race-, and gender-matched population.

Dubin-Johnson syndrome: A rare autosomal recessive genetic disorder of hepatic bilirubin clearance leading to increased levels of conjugated bilirubin in the blood stream and the clinical presentation of jaundice, with possible hepatomegaly and right upper quadrant discomfort usually occurring in the teenage years. It is caused by a mutation in the gene coding for human canalicular multispecific organic anion transporter protein, which is also called *multidrug resistance protein 2*, impacting ATP-dependent transport across the canalicular membrane of hepatocytes. The course is generally benign and is not associated with liver fibrosis or cirrhosis. Pregnancy and hormonal contraceptives may exacerbate the defect.

ductal dilation: Increase in the diameter of a main duct or branch of a bile or pancreatic duct usually implying pathologic obstruction or narrowing. It can be detected by ultrasound, CT, or MRI and is usually caused by choledocholithiasis, lymphadenopathy, or malignant obstruction. Treatment includes endoscopic retrograde cholangiopancreatography-based interventions or interventional or surgical decompression if no easily reversible cause is identified.

duct of Santorini: *Another term for* accessory pancreatic duct.

duct of Wirsung: *Another term for* main pancreatic duct.

ductopenia: A decreased number or complete absence of bile ducts or ductules on liver biopsy histology. It is generally associated with chronic rejection in a liver transplant biopsy or advanced stage primary biliary cirrhosis in a native liver. Drug-induced liver injury may also present with ductopenia.

ducts of Luschka: Small branches of intrahepatic bile ducts that run from the hepatic parenchyma directly into the right hepatic duct, common hepatic duct, or the gallbladder bed. This anomaly can be a source of postoperative bile leak if not recognized during a cholecystectomy. A clinically significant leak is rare from these small radicles, but endoscopic stenting or surgical intervention may be necessary if present.

duct-to-duct anastomosis: The most common biliary connection made in liver transplantation in which a connection between the native bile duct remnant is made to the donor bile duct rather than to a loop of the small intestine (*see* Roux-en-Y hepaticojejunostomy).

ductular proliferation: A histologic finding on liver biopsy that occurs in the setting of chronic biliary obstruction whereby the formation of immature biliary structures, called bile ductules, is promoted as a response to inadequate biliary drainage.

ductule: A small intrahepatic portion of the biliary system located in the portal triad that functions to direct bile from the bile canaliculi of the hepatocytes to the larger intrahepatic bile ducts.

dumping syndrome: Rapid emptying of gastric contents into the small intestine that can occur after partial gastrectomy, bariatric surgery, or vagotomy. The syndrome includes abdominal cramping, nausea, diaphoresis, and palpitations. Hypotension and tachycardia may also be present on vital sign measurements. Treatment includes reducing intake of simple sugars; increasing intake of fiber, protein, and complex carbohydrates; eating smaller meals; and separating the consumption of liquids and solids by 30 minutes.

duodenal bulb: The first segment of the duodenum, located just distal to the pylorus. It is also a common site for peptic ulcers and Brunner's gland hyperplasia.

duodenal diverticulum: Outpouching of the mucosa and submucosa, usually on the medial side of the duodenum near the ampulla. The duodenum is the most common site for small intestine diverticula. It is a rare cause of upper GI bleeding. More commonly, its presence may make ERCP cannulation of the ampulla more difficult and increase the risk of ERCP-related duodenal perforation.

duodenal duplication cyst: A rare congenital cystic formation on the duodenal wall composed of smooth muscle and GI mucosa. Its most common site is posterior to the first and second portion of the duodenum. It can be clinically silent but can also be a cause of partial gastric outlet obstruction or bleeding (due to it containing heterotopic gastric mucosa) and can become infected.

duodenal stenosis: Narrowing of the lumen of the duodenum that can be secondary to a variety of processes, including annular pancreas, developmental anomalies, pancreatic cancer, or fibrosis from severe peptic ulcer disease. Diagnosis is made radiographically using a barium study or by endoscopy. Treatment includes endoscopic or interventional radiology-guided stenting or dilatation or surgical bypass.

duodenal switch surgery: A type of weight loss surgery, also known as biliopancreatic diversion with duodenal switch, that accomplishes weight loss by inducing malabsorption. It is an effective surgery for weight loss but is not commonly performed due to the high risk of vitamin and mineral deficiencies associated with malabsorption, difficult surgical technique, and higher associated morbidity and mortality.

duodenal ulcer: Localized erosion of the duodenal mucosa, most often due to infection with *H pylori* or NSAID use. Endoscopy and radiologic testing can be used to make the diagnosis. Treatment is the elimination of NSAIDs, initiation of proton pump inhibitors, and eradication of *H pylori,* if present. Malignant duodenal ulcers are rare and less common than malignant gastric ulcers; therefore, biopsies are not mandatory.

duodenal varices: A dilated submucosal venous structure in the duodenum caused by portal hypertension that is an infrequent cause of upper GI bleeding. Treatment includes band ligation, injection sclerotherapy, and reversal of portal hypertension (eg, transjugular intrahepatic portosystemic shunt or liver transplantation).

duodenum: The first section of the small intestine, beginning distal to the pylorus and ending at the duodenojejunal junction, that is supported by the ligament of Treitz (suspensory ligament of the duodenum). The duodenum can be divided into 4 parts: superior, descending, inferior, and ascending. Its primary roles include digestion via mixing of gastric contents, bile, and pancreatic enzymes, as well as the absorption of important nutrients, including iron.

duplex ultrasonography: A standard imaging modality using color flow dopplers during ultrasound testing to evaluate blood flow in the veins or arteries in various places in the body. It is a commonly used test for the diagnosis of deep vein thrombosis but can be used on the abdomen to evaluate for portal or hepatic vein thrombosis, renal artery stenosis, and celiac artery stenosis.

Dupuytren's contracture: A slowly progressive idiopathic disease that causes thickening of the palmar fascia resulting in an inability to extend the fourth and fifth digits. It is commonly seen in alcoholics and patients with cirrhosis. The pathogenesis is unknown. Treatment is surgical or conservative if no functional limitations are present.

dyschezia: Infrequent, painful bowel movements that may be caused by pelvic floor dysfunction or impaired relaxation of the muscles of defecation. In infants, it usually resolves spontaneously. In adults, treatment is aimed at improving the cause of pelvic floor dysfunction.

dyspepsia: Pain, burning, or discomfort in the epigastric area often caused by peptic ulcer disease, GERD, food intolerances, or gastritis. Upper endoscopy and CT scan may be used in the diagnostic algorithm. Treatment is aimed at the underlying cause and may include acid suppression, treatment of *H pylori* infection, and dietary modification.

dysphagia: Difficulty swallowing solid foods or liquids. Many etiologies exist, including GI motility disorders, anatomic GI disease, and neurologic insult. Endoscopy and barium esophagram are first-line diagnostic tests. Treatment is aimed at the cause of dysphagia but could include endoscopic dilatation, medication, diet modification, surgery, or even chemotherapy or radiation therapy if a malignant etiology is detected; *see* Appendix 13.

dysplasia: Preneoplastic disordered growth of cells representing a disrupted growth regulation that is a high-risk condition for cancer. In GI, this most often refers to colonic adenomas and Barrett's esophagus, which are dysplastic conditions that can progress to cancer if not treated or removed.

dysplasia-associated lesions or masses (DALMs): Preneoplastic areas located within a segment of inflamed colonic mucosa in patients with IBD. The detection of this lesion is difficult and often encountered with surveillance biopsies. If present, colectomy is recommended because it is high risk for cancer formation.

early virologic response: A phrase used to define a decrease in hepatitis C viral ribonucleic acid (RNA) load by more than 2 logs after 12 weeks of pegylated interferon-based therapy. Patients who fail to achieve early virologic response are likely to have nonresponse to treatment, and treatment discontinuation is recommended due to predicted futility. Complete early virologic response means that the virus is completely suppressed by 12 weeks of treatment.

Echinococcus: A type of tapeworm whose primary hosts are dogs, and intermediate hosts are sheep, cattle, and humans when inadvertent ingestion of the *Echinococcus* eggs occurs. Ingestion by humans can lead to the formation of hydatid cysts (well-defined, large cystic lesions) often occurring in the liver. The cysts are usually asymptomatic, but hepatic cysts can rupture and cause cholangitis, biliary colic, pancreatitis, or, rarely, portal hypertension as a result of the pressure effect on the perihepatic vasculature. Serologies exist to aid in the diagnosis. Albendazole is the preferred anti-helminthic agent used for treatment.

ectopic pancreas: A congenital anomaly of abnormally located pancreatic tissue most commonly found in the submucosa of the stomach, duodenum, small intestine, or Meckel's diverticulum. It usually has little clinical significance but rarely can be a cause of abdominal pain.

ectopic varices: Presence of dilated submucosal venous structures associated with portal hypertension outside of the esophagus or stomach, such as in the duodenum or jejunum. They are a rare cause of GI bleeding and may be difficult to diagnose because they are outside the view of traditional upper endoscopy and

Fenkel JM, ed.
Quick Reference Dictionary for GI and Hepatology (pp 60-68).
© 2014 Taylor & Francis Group.

colonoscopy. Treatment is aimed at the reversal of portal hypertension (eg, transjugular intrahepatic portosystemic shunt or liver transplantation).

efferent loop syndrome: A rare complication of gastric surgery, usually occurring in the first few postoperative weeks, in which patients may experience nausea, cramping, abdominal distention relieved by vomiting, and bilious emesis. It is usually caused by an internal hernia or intussusception and requires surgical treatment.

electrohydraulic lithotripsy: A technique used to dissolve stones in the GI and genitourinary tract using a probe that functions to induce a spark between two electrodes at the end of the probe, creating a hydraulic shockwave. In GI, this treatment is a laborious one reserved for bile or pancreatic duct stones that fail conventional endoscopic treatment. It is used during an ERCP.

emesis: The medical term for vomiting. Other medical terms include this root: hematemesis (vomiting blood) and hyperemesis (frequent vomiting).

endometriosis: Benign endometrial glands and stroma found outside the uterus that can cause cyclic, catamenial, abdominal pain, and infertility. Most commonly seen on the ovaries but may also appear in other locations, including the fallopian tubes, uterine ligament, pouch of Douglas, rectovaginal pouch, bladder wall, rectosigmoid colon, and umbilicus.

endoscope: A medical device consisting of a flexible, lighted fiberoptic tube that allows for visualization of the GI tract by a gastroenterologist. The term *endoscope* refers to the instrument used in upper endoscopy and colonoscopy.

endoscopic band ligation: A method used to treat esophageal varices that uses an endoscope and high-pressure rubber bands to tie off varices. Used to treat acute variceal bleeding and for the prevention of variceal bleeding in large varices or varices with high-risk stigmata for bleeding.

endoscopic cystduodenostomy: An endoscopic method for surgical drainage of a pancreatic pseudocyst that creates a connection between the cyst cavity and the duodenum, allowing drainage to occur via internally placed stents.

endoscopic cystgastrostomy: An endoscopic method for surgical drainage of a pancreatic pseudocyst by creating a connection between the cyst cavity and the posterior wall of the stomach, allowing drainage to occur via internally placed stents.

endoscopic mucosal resection: An endoscopic technique used to remove dysplastic mucosa or sessile polyps (flat polyps) by elevating the lesion away from the submucosa using banding or submucosal injection or by applying a traction method before removing it. This is a common technique in the management of dysplastic Barrett's esophagus and flat colonic adenomas.

endoscopic pancreatic necrosectomy: A technique for minimally invasive debridement of necrotic pancreatic tissue and walled-off pancreatic necrosis after complicated acute pancreatitis. A small hole is created in the stomach wall and an endoscope is driven through it into the area of necrosis, where suction and various endoscopic tools can aid in the removal of infected tissue and fluid. It is not yet the gold standard treatment; however, it may have improved outcomes over an open surgical technique.

endoscopic retrograde cholangiopancreatography (ERCP): A procedure that involves cannulation of the bile duct to perform diagnostic imaging of the biliary or pancreatic ducts or to allow for therapeutic intervention, such as stenting or stone extraction. The major diagnostic uses are for the diagnosis of primary sclerosing cholangitis, cholangiocarcinoma, and sphincter of Oddi dysfunction. Its major therapeutic uses include stone extraction, sphincterotomy, stent placement, and biliary brush cytology and biopsy. The major risks associated with the procedure include pancreatitis (range, 5% to 10%), bleeding (less than 1%), and perforation (less than 1%).

endoscopic retrograde pancreatography: Cannulation of the pancreatic duct during ERCP for the purpose of diagnostic imaging or management of pancreatic duct strictures or stones. Endoscopic retrograde pancreatography can be used in the setting of chronic pancreatitis to stent the duct, perform a minor papillotomy, or aid in the diagnosis of pancreatic ductal adenocarcinoma. Risks are similar to ERCP but also include pancreatic duct leak (less than 1%).

endoscopic ultrasound (EUS): An imaging technique that uses a high-frequency ultrasound tranducer on the tip of an endoscope to obtain high-resolution images of the GI tract and adjacent structures, including the pancreas, liver, and regional lymph nodes. A fine needle may be introduced through the scope to directly sample an area of abnormality identified by the EUS.

endoscopy: A general term for a procedure that uses either a flexible tube with an illuminated lens at the tip or a small ingestible camera to visualize a cavity within the body. This includes laryngoscopy, bronchoscopy, esophagogastroduodenoscopy, and colonoscopy.

endoscopy unit: A free-standing surgicenter or part of a hospital dedicated specifically to performing endoscopies that has trained endoscopy nurses and contains endoscopic equipment.

Entamoeba: An intestinal protozoan parasite that can cause amebic colitis and amebic liver abscess in humans. Infection usually occurs in endemic areas such as Central and South America, Africa, and India but can rarely occur after solid organ transplantation. Treatment is with metronidazole or tinidazole, followed by paromomycin.

Enterobius vermicularis: A helminth parasite found in the United States, commonly known as pinworm, that is acquired via ingestion of parasite eggs. The presenting symptom is usually nocturnal perianal itching from female pinworm deposition of eggs on the perianal skin. The diagnosis is made when removal of cellophane tape that was applied to the perianal area reveals eggs. Everyone in close contact with the patient should be treated with mebendazole or albendazole for 3 to 7 days.

enterochromaffin-like (ECL) cell: A type of enteroendocrine cell found in the parietal glands of the fundus and body of the stomach and in the mucosa of the intestines. ECL cells function in secreting histamine to help regulate gastric acid secretion and intestinal motility.

Enterococcus: A gram positive aerobic species of bacteria often colonizing the GI tract that is a frequent cause of hospital acquired infections, with *Enterococcus faecalis* being the most common species. *Enterococcus* is especially problematic because of the amount of antibiotic resistance in this species, notably vancomycin-resistant *Enterococcus*.

enteroscopy: A specific type of endoscopy used to visualize the small intestine. Due to its extensive length, visualization of the small intestine endoscopically is challenging. The endoscopic techniques used to visualize the small bowel include push enteroscopy, device-assisted enteroscopy, and wireless capsule enteroscopy.

enterovesical fistula: An abnormal connection between the bladder and the GI tract that usually presents as recurrent urinary tract infection and pneumaturia (air in the urine). The fistula can be caused by congenital anomaly, Crohn's disease, complicated diverticulitis, malignant invasion, or surgical complication or as a result of trauma. Treatment is usually surgical, although the fistula may close with biologic or immunomodulator therapy in patients with Crohn's disease.

eosinophilic esophagitis: An intrinsic cause of esophageal dysphagia usually seen in children or young adults. It presents as intermittent dysphagia to solid foods or as an acute food bolus impaction. The diagnosis is made by an endoscopy that shows multiple esophageal rings and linear furrows, as well as by esophageal biopsies that show more than 15 eosinophils per high powered field in the mucosa. Topical steroids, such as fluticasone or budesonide, are used for treatment. In children, elimination diets are also used to identify potential food triggers. Food triggers are less common in adult presentations of the disease.

eosinophilic gastroenteritis: A rare disease characterized by eosinophilic infiltration of the GI luminal wall to variable depths (mucosal, muscular, or serosal) at multiple sites throughout the GI tract. It most often affects the stomach or the small intestine; however, presentation is variable and dependent on the depth of infiltration. A biopsy of the GI tract is needed to make the diagnosis. It is usually responsive to treatment with corticosteroids.

Eovist: A type of MRI contrast agent that is useful in the diagnosis of focal liver lesions, the characteristics of which include hepatocyte uptake and biliary excretion; *also known as* gadoxetate disodium.

epigallocatechin-3-gallate (EGCG): A metabolite found in green tea that is thought to have antitumor effects, such as the inhibition of cell growth, reduction of COX-2 expression, induction of apoptosis, and anti-oxidant, anti-fibrotic, and anti-inflammatory properties. At high doses, it can be hepatotoxic. Green tea is hypothesized to have a protective effect in several diseases but is not yet recommended for prevention.

episcleritis: Inflammation of the thin layer between the conjunctiva and sclera of the eye manifesting as a painless, localized area of redness with dilated vessels. This is a common extraintestinal condition associated with ulcerative colitis.

epithelioid hemangioendothelioma: A rare vascular tumor of the liver characterized as highly vascular, multifocal, and endothelial in origin. It is often asymptomatic but can cause abdominal pain, nausea, and portal hypertension if a large portion of the hepatic parenchyma is involved. Liver transplantation offers the greatest chance of survival and disease-free survival.

erythema nodosum: Warm, red, and tender nodules that develop on the anterior shins and are commonly associated with IBD but may also be found in other inflammatory conditions.

Escherichia coli: A species of food-borne, gram-negative bacteria that includes both benign and highly virulent strains. It is a major component in the normal flora of the GI tract; however, many strains can also cause diarrheal illness, pneumonia, bacteremia, and peritonitis. In addition, it is the most common cause of urinary tract infections.

esophageal adenocarcinoma: A type of primary esophageal cancer that is now the most common type of esophageal cancer in the United States. It primarily develops in the distal one-third of the esophagus, usually in the setting of dysplastic Barrett's esophagus, which is the strongest risk factor in its development.

esophageal diverticulum: An outpouching of the esophageal wall that can be true or false. A true diverticulum contains all three layers of the esophagus, whereas a false diverticulum only contains mucosa and submucosa. It may present with dysphagia or halitosis. Surgical treatment may be required depending on the severity of symptoms and location.

esophageal intramural pseudodiverticulosis: Multiple small out-pouchings of the esophagus usually found on barium swallow. These are actually not true diverticula but rather represent the dilated ducts of esophageal submucosal glands. They are often associated with chronic candidal infection and may be a risk factor for the formation of esophageal strictures, esophageal cancer, or esophageal motility disorders.

esophageal motility testing: A diagnostic procedure used to help identify motility disorders of the esophagus and upper GI tract. In this procedure, a thin, flexible catheter is passed through the nose into the lower esophagus and stomach. The patient is instructed to swallow so that the pressure of esophageal con-tractions is measured through the catheter. This information can then be used to diagnose specific motility disorders and initiate a management strategy. Motility tests include standard and high-resolution manometry.

esophageal perforation: Transmural rupture of the esophagus most commonly caused by iatrogenic instrumentation (ie, endoscopy, dilatation) but can also be caused by prolonged esophageal obstruction, severe vomiting (Boerhaave's syn-drome), external trauma, severe eosinophilic esophagitis, and, rarely, ulcer disease. Treatment includes nothing-by-mouth status, broad-spectrum antibiotics, and surgical intervention.

esophageal ring: Circumferential muscular bands of benign tissue usually located in the lower esophagus that can cause dyspha-gia. They are typically composed of hypertrophied muscle. Schatzki's rings are a type of esophageal ring composed of mucosa and submucosa. Endoscopic dilatation is the first-line therapy for symptomatic rings. Asymptomatic rings do not usu-ally require intervention.

esophageal squamous cell carcinoma: The most common type of esophageal cancer worldwide, usually occurring in the middle one-third of the esophagus. Tobacco and alcohol abuse signifi-cantly increase the risk of obtaining this disease.

esophageal stent: An artificial tube (usually composed of a metal alloy) that is deployed into the area of esophageal stricture during endoscopy. The stent expands, embeds itself into the surrounding tissue, and restores patency of the esophagus. This treatment has been used primarily as a palliative treatment for malignant dysphagia but may also be used in a variety of other diseases, including benign esophageal strictures and tracheo-esophageal fistulas.

esophageal stricture: A narrowing of the esophageal lumen that presents as dysphagia, acute food bolus, or foreign body impaction. Stricture can be secondary to intrinsic causes, such as chronic acid reflux or esophageal adenocarcinoma, or extrinsic causes, such as mediastinal lymphadenopathy. Treatment is targeted at the etiology of the stricture but often includes endoscopic dilatation or stent placement in combination with acid suppressive medications.

esophageal ulcer: An erosion of the mucosal lining in the esophagus, which is an uncommon cause of esophageal bleeding. It can be secondary to esophagitis or iatrogenic from sclerotherapy, bisphosphonates, and other treatments. Viruses, including herpes simplex, HIV, and cytomegalovirus, can also cause esophageal ulcers, and biopsies are helpful in determining the inciting etiology.

esophageal web: Congenital or inflammatory abnormality composed of a thin membrane of squamous epithelium usually found protruding from the anterior wall of the cervical esophagus. It can be a cause of esophageal dysphagia and is associated with Plummer-Vinson syndrome.

esophagectomy: Surgical excision of a portion of or the entire esophagus, usually as a treatment for esophageal cancer. Available techniques include laparoscopic, open, and transhiatal approaches.

esophagitis: Inflammation of the esophagus, which can be nonerosive or erosive. There are many etiologies, including acid-peptic, caustic, infectious, and noninfectious causes. If acid related, histamine receptor antagonists and proton pump inhibitors are commonly used to help heal the inflammation.

esophagus: A muscular tube connecting the pharynx to the stomach whose principal role is to transport food into the stomach for digestion by active and passive/reflexive means.

ethiodol: An oil-based contrast agent used in chemoembolization surveillance imaging procedures to help monitor response. It is also used as a contrast medium for hysterosalpingography and lymphangiography and can be used as an additive to cyanoacrylate for use in gastric variceal obturation procedures.

evacuation proctography: *Another term for* barium defecography; *see* defecography.

extended rapid virologic response: Undetectable viral load at weeks 4 and 12 in a patient undergoing anti-viral treatment for hepatitis C. Patients who achieve this response are often eligible for shortened duration or response-guided therapy and have a higher predicted rate of sustained virologic response following treatment completion.

external anal sphincter: A circular skeletal muscle located at the distal end of the anal canal, which is under voluntary control. This is one of the major components of the anal sphincter complex, along with the internal anal sphincter and puborectalis, and functions to maintain stool continence.

extracorporeal shockwave lithotripsy: A technique in which high-energy sound waves are used to fragment a stone in the genitourinary system or the GI tract from outside the body. Gallbladder stones respond less well to this technique, but it can be used in difficult cases where other treatment modalities have been unsuccessful or where cholecystectomy is contraindicated. It is also commonly used for minor orthopedic injuries, such as tennis elbow or plantar fasciitis.

extrahepatic: Occurring or existing outside the liver. This term is used to describe the location of a finding in the bile ducts, particularly choledocholithiasis or strictures. Extrahepatic abnormalities are often more endoscopically accessible during therapeutic intervention than intrahepatic lesions.

familial adenomatous polyposis (FAP): An autosomal dominant inherited colon cancer disorder most often caused by a germ-line mutation in the adenomatous polyposis coli tumor suppressor gene on chromosome 5 that causes mutations in DNA mismatch repair genes. The disease is characterized by the development of colon polyps that will progress until the colon is entirely covered with polyps, with colon cancer an inevitable consequence by age 50 years.

familial Mediterranean fever (FMF): An autosomal recessive inherited disease that presents as recurrent episodes of fever, joint pain, and abdominal pain. Abdominal pain is frequently the presenting symptom and can mimic acute appendicitis. These patients are at a high risk for developing small bowel obstructions and systemic amyloidosis.

fatty liver: Diffuse macro- or microvesicular steatosis present in the liver. It can be caused by alcohol or nonalcoholic fatty liver disease (NAFLD). Usually, patients are asymptomatic, with mild elevations in their liver enzymes. Approximately 10% of patients with a fatty liver will have inflammation associated with the fat causing steatohepatitis, which puts them at risk for developing cirrhosis and liver failure in the future.

fecal fat: A diagnostic test for steatorrhea that can be a quantitative or qualitative analysis. Fecal fat is increased in malabsorption diseases and pancreatic insufficiency. A Sudan stain is used to accentuate fat on the slide.

fecal immunohistochemistry test (FIT): A type of stool-based test used for CRC screening that requires the patient to collect multiple stool samples. Fluorescently tagged antibodies specific for a protein on red blood cells are then applied to the samples to detect blood in the stool. It has been demonstrated to be more accurate than guaiac testing but not as accurate as colonoscopy for the detection of CRC.

fecal impaction: Partial or complete obstruction of the rectal vault by stool. It can present as abdominal pain, distention, nausea, vomiting, and paradoxical diarrhea (as liquid stool overflows around the impaction). Treatment includes manual disimpaction, intestinal decompression if complete obstruction is present, laxatives, and stool softeners.

fecal incontinence: Involuntary expulsion of fecal material that can range from unintentional flatus to complete expulsion of the contents in the rectal vault. Anorectal manometry can aid in the diagnosis and treatment planning.

fecal occult blood test (FOBT): A screening tool for CRC that detects the presence of nonvisible blood in the stool. There are two types: guaiac test and fecal immunohistochemistry test. Both tests require patients do a home collection of multiple stool samples, and neither are very sensitive.

fecal osmotic gap: The difference between the measured osmolality of the stool and the estimated osmolality of stool, which should be less than 50 mosm/kg. An increase in osmotic gap indicates that diarrhea is due to an osmotically active substance. The equation to calculate fecal osmotic gap involves subtracting twice the fecal concentrations of sodium and potassium from 290 mosm/kg, the osmolality of stool in the body: $290 - 2[(Na+) + (K+)]$.

fecaluria: The presence of fecal material in urine. This symptom is highly suggestive of an enterovesical or colovesical fistula.

feeding jejunostomy: Placement of a feeding tube directly into the jejunum to provide enteral nutrition in patients who cannot tolerate gastric feedings or those who have had complications of tube feeding aspiration with gastric feeding.

feeding tube: A device used to provide enteral access for nutrition to patients unable to eat or drink by mouth due to neurologic or GI dysfunction. This phrase can refer to any of the following devices: nasogastric tube, nasojejunal tube, PEG, percutaneous endoscopic jejunostomy, or surgical jejunostomy.

feline esophagus: An endoscopic finding of eosinophilic esophagitis; *also known as* a corrugated or ringed esophagus.

ferritin: A protein that functions in intracellular iron storage. Levels of ferritin fluctuate congruently with iron levels in the body; therefore, ferritin is a good marker of iron overload or deficiency. However, levels may also be elevated by any acute phase reaction.

fetor hepaticus: The musty breath odor of patients with advanced cirrhosis.

fever: An elevated body temperature that is often a marker of infection, inflammation, or malignancy. A patient with a fever often feels hot and sweaty, or may have chills and experience shivers. Identifying the source of the fever is the first step in knowing whether treatment is required. Acetaminophen or ibuprofen is often used to treat fever when a clear cause is not identified or for symptom relief; *also called* pyrexia.

fiber: A nondigestable structural component of plant cell walls found in fruits, vegetables, oat, barley, dried beans, and rye. It is also a medical therapy to increase stool caliber or bulk in patients with chronic diarrhea. When taken in higher doses, it draws water into the colonic lumen and may be a medical therapy for constipation.

fibrolamellar hepatocellular carcinoma: A rare variant of liver cancer that is not associated with hepatitis, cirrhosis, or alpha fetoprotein production. It usually presents in young adults as multifocal liver tumors with metastases and often is not responsive to chemotherapy.

Fibroscan: Device developed by Echosens that uses ultrasound waves to quantify liver stiffness to estimate the amount of liver fibrosis; *also known as* transient elastography.

FibroSure: A blood test manufactured by LabCorp used to estimate the degree of fibrosis in patients with hepatitis C and other chronic liver diseases. It includes haptoglobin levels, bilirubin, gamma-glutamyl transpeptidase, apo-lipoprotein A-l, and α2-macroglobulin, although in variable ratios depending on the producer. This test, whose result ranges from 0 to 1, has a high negative predictive value but is not as accurate as the score approaches a value of 1.

fibrovascular polyp of the esophagus: A rare, benign growth located at the upper esophageal sphincter that can cause asphyxiation and dysphagia. Endoscopic or surgical resection is curative.

fine-needle aspiration (FNA): A method of sampling tissue through a small needle guided into a lesion, resulting in a cellular suspension that can be analyzed for the presence of malignancy or other etiologies. It can be performed percutaneously or endoscopically and is commonly used in the diagnostic workup of pancreatic lesions via EUS.

fissure: A linear, sharply defined erosion of epidermis and dermis or mucosa. In the GI tract, they are most commonly found in the anal area, often occurring as a result of constipation and straining.

fistula: An abnormal communication between two epithelium-lined structures that can include organs, skin, or blood vessels. They can occur as a complication of Crohn's disease, surgery, or radiation treatment. Symptoms and treatment vary depending on which two structures are connected.

flat spot: An endoscopically visualized area of pigmentation at the base of a peptic ulcer. The finding is suggestive of a recently bleeding ulcer, is associated with a low risk of re-bleeding, and does not require any further endoscopic intervention.

flatus: Air or gas that is expelled from or generated by the GI tract.

flexible sigmoidoscopy: A procedure similar to a colonoscopy, but a shorter scope is used, allowing for visualization of the left colon only. The standard procedure does not require sedation, and enemas are used instead of a complete bowel preparation. Patients who are found to have polyps on this examination must then undergo a colonoscopy to provide visualization of the entire colon.

florid duct lesion: A histopathologic feature of primary biliary cirrhosis in which the bile duct is infiltrated by lymphocyte and plasma cells, forming necrosis and a granulomatous reaction.

fluoroscopy: An imaging technique that uses continuous radiographic imaging to obtain a real time video of a part of the body. Uses within gastroenterology include GI motility evaluation, ERCP, and luminal stent placement.

focal nodular hyperplasia: A benign lesion of the liver that is more prevalent in women. The histopathologic features are characterized by a single, well-circumscribed area of hyperplastic hepatocytes surrounding a central scar. It often has a distinct radiographic appearance, with the central scar visible on imaging; *also called* focal cirrhosis.

folate: A water-soluble vitamin necessary for many human functions, including DNA synthesis. Foods that contain the highest amount of folate are liver, greens, nuts, and beans. Alcoholics are particularly susceptible to folate deficiency and should receive supplements.

food bolus impaction: Food that causes an obstruction in the esophagus requiring urgent endoscopic removal or advancement to the stomach. Certain conditions, including eosinophilic esophagitis and untreated GERD, predispose individuals to food impaction.

foreign body: An item that does not naturally belong within the body. A foreign body can become impacted in the GI tract, most commonly the esophagus, and require endoscopic or surgical retrieval to prevent perforation and aspiration.

fossa: A shallow depression on a surface (eg, gallbladder fossa).

free hepatic venous pressure (FHVP): The pressure measured within the hepatic vein or inferior vena cava before a wedged measurement is taken during a transjugular liver study. Elevated free hepatic pressure can be observed in patients with right heart failure, pulmonary hypertension, and Budd-Chiari syndrome.

French: A unit of measurement, usually seen as "French catheter," that refers to the French scale of catheter measurement where 1 Fr = 0.33 mm. It is a measurement of circumference not diameter; therefore, increasing French size indicates a larger catheter diameter. This is contrary to needle-gauge size, where an increasing gauge corresponds with a smaller diameter needle.

Frey procedure: A surgical procedure for pancreatic head-predominant chronic pancreatitis that involves removing the diseased portion and performing a lateral pancreaticojejunostomy (connecting the pancreatic duct to a loop of jejunum).

fulminant liver failure: The rapid development of coagulation abnormalities and encephalopathy in a patient with previously normal liver function. Etiologies include acetaminophen or other drug-induced liver injury, autoimmune hepatitis, Wilson's disease, amanita mushroom poisoning, or herbal- or dietary supplement-induced liver injury. The Kings College criteria are helpful in determining which patients will recover and which patients will need a liver transplantation. Patients with this condition receive priority status on the liver transplant wait list.

functional constipation: *See* chronic constipation.

functional dyspepsia: *See* non-ulcer dyspepsia.

fundic gland polyps: Most common type of gastric gland polyp. They have a low malignant potential, are usually asymptomatic, and do not typically require excision. Use of proton pump inhibitors can increase their formation.

fundus: The superior portion of the stomach located between the cardia and the body.

fungal esophagitis: Inflammation of the esophagus caused by a fungus, most often *Candida albicans*. Usually, it is only seen in patients who are immunocompromised, unless an underlying motility disorder causing stasis exists. Treatment includes anti-fungal medication and restoration of immune function as best as possible.

gadolinium: A common component of MRI intravenous contrast agents. Its use in patients with chronic kidney disease has been associated with a rare condition called nephrogenic systemic fibrosis and, as such, caution of its use is advised in patients with chronic kidney disease.

gallbladder: An organ that functions to store and secrete bile produced by the liver. Its primary function is to secrete stored bile into the duodenum once stimulated by cholecystokinin. Bile aids in digestion.

gallbladder cancer: A malignant tumor of the gallbladder (typically an adenocarcinoma) that is more prevalent in women then men. Risk factors include gallstones, porcelain gallbladder, and large adenomatous polyps of the gallbladder. Surgery is the only potentially curative treatment, and prognosis is poor if the malignancy is unresectable.

gallbladder sludge: An asymptomatic condition of the gallbladder that may arise from bile stasis and bile supersaturation with cholesterol or calcium bilirubinate. It is associated with the development of gallstones and may be a cause of acute pancreatitis.

gallstone: Concretions that form within the gallbladder, *also referred to as* cholelithiasis, that are usually composed of cholesterol or bile pigment. Gallstones can be asymptomatic or present with postprandial right upper quadrant pain. The standard diagnostic procedure is a right upper quadrant ultrasound. If symptomatic, cholecystectomy is the standard treatment; *see* Appendix 26.

Fenkel JM, ed.
Quick Reference Dictionary for GI and Hepatology (pp 75-83).
© 2014 Taylor & Francis Group.

gallstone ileus: An uncommon cause of a small bowel obstruction due to a large gallstone that is impacted in the intestinal lumen, most commonly at the ileocecal valve. The stone usually creates a cholecystoduodenal fistula as a means for its passage into the GI tract because it is too large to pass through the ampulla into the duodenum.

gallstone pancreatitis: Acute pancreatitis caused by a gallstone, typically by obstructing the ampulla of Vater. Treatment is supportive and includes intravenous fluids, bowel rest, analgesia, and eventual reintroduction of low-fat food once the acute inflammation is improved. Cholecystectomy and biliary sphincterotomy are options to prevent recurrent gallstone pancreatitis.

Gardner's syndrome: A phenotypic subtype of FAP that includes the classic intestinal adenomas with desmoid tumors, bony tumors, dental abnormalities, congenital hypertrophy of the retinal pigment epithelium, and mesenteric fibromatosis.

gastric antral vascular ectasia: A vascular lesion that consists of multiple dilated vessels radiating from the pylorus that, when seen by endoscope, resembles the skin of a watermelon; *also referred to as* watermelon stomach. It can be a cause of acute or chronic GI bleeding and is often treated with argon plasma coagulation to the affected areas of the stomach and iron supplementation if iron-deficiency anemia is present.

gastric bezoar: *See* bezoar.

gastric diverticulum: A rare type of outpouching (diverticulum), the most common of which is a false diverticulum and involves the mucosa and submucosa only. It is most often located on the lesser curvature near the esophagogastric junction. A less common type is an intramural diverticulum on the greater curvature that has mucosa projecting into the muscularis.

gastric duplication cyst: A congenital anomaly of a noncommunicating cystic mass that shares a wall with the stomach and is found along the greater curvature or posterior wall. It resembles a second stomach in that it contains all gastric wall layers, as well as gastric and pancreatic mucosa. EUS may be useful in its evaluation.

gastric emptying scan: An imaging study used to evaluate the rate of gastric emptying by tracing the progression of radionucleotide labeled meals over several hours and measuring the percentage emptied. In a normal patient, 50% of the ingested meal should be emptied in 2 hours. If more than 50% remains after 2 hours, then the patient is diagnosed with delayed gastric emptying or gastroparesis.

gastric intestinal metaplasia: Replacement of gastric epithelium with features of intestinal epithelium in the form of columnar cells, goblet cells, or paneth cells. It may represent an increased risk for gastric cancer. The effectiveness of surveillance strategies is unclear, but surveillance is often pursued by gastroenterologists.

gastric lavage: A treatment used to empty the stomach of its contents, most commonly used for GI hemorrhage or toxic ingestion. The procedure requires placement of a large lumen nasogastric or orogastric tube, administration of small amounts of room temperature tap water or saline through the tube, and withdrawal of the same fluid. This process is continued until the lavage fluid returns clear. The return of blood on lavage suggests an active upper GI bleeding, and an urgent endoscopy is recommended.

gastric outlet obstruction: Partial or complete blockage at the level of the pylorus or duodenal bulb that prevents complete emptying of the stomach. The most common symptoms are early satiety, nausea, weight loss, and emesis of partially digested food hours after eating. It is typically due to malignant obstruction or severe peptic ulcer disease. Acid suppression, nasogastric tube decompression, and surgery are the mainstays of treatment. Endoscopic stent placement and venting gastrostomy may also play a role in its management.

gastric pacemaker: A treatment for refractory gastoparesis that uses an implantable pacemaker to deliver low-energy electrical currents to stimulate gastric contractions and improve emptying. It may also be referred to as gastric electrical stimulation.

gastric polyp: Benign growths in the stomach that can be classified as adenomatous, hamartomatous, heterotopic, hyperplastic, or inflammatory. The most common are hyperplastic polyps. Endoscopic targeted biopsies can distinguish between the different types.

gastric ulcer: Localized erosion of the gastric mucosa, most often due to infection with *H pylori* or the use of NSAIDs. The mainstay of treatment is acid suppression and mucosal healing with proton pump inhibitors. Biopsy should be performed to exclude malignancy and to assess for *H pylori*. If presenting as bleeding, endoscopic evaluation is standard and therapeutic maneuvers can often be performed to decrease the risk of rebleeding. Follow-up EGD is recommended in patients diagnosed with gastric ulcers to ensure healing because gastric ulcers occasionally represent early gastric cancer, a diagnosis one does not wish to miss.

gastric volvulus: Twisting of the stomach around an axis—either organoaxial (long direction) or mesenteroaxial (short direction). Classically, it presents with Borchardt's triad. Treatment is surgery.

gastrin: A hormone produced by G cells in the stomach that stimulates gastric acid secretion and promotes proliferation of the gastric mucosa.

gastrinoma: A gastrin-secreting tumor that causes hypersecretion of acid leading to severe peptic ulcer disease, diarrhea, and abdominal pain. It can be sporadic or associated with multiple endocrine neoplasia type 1; *see also* Zollinger-Ellison syndrome.

gastrinoma triangle: The typical location of a gastrinoma, this anatomical space is bordered superiorly by the confluence of the common bile duct and cystic duct, inferiorly by the second and third portion of the duodenum, and medically by the pancreatic neck–body junction.

gastritis: Inflammation of the stomach mucosa that can be acute or chronic and infectious or noninfectious. *H pylori* infection, NSAID use, and alcohol consumption are common causes. The diagnosis is usually made by endoscopy with biopsies. Treatment includes proton pump inhibitors, eradication of *H pylori* infection, cessation of offending agents, and antiemetics if nausea is associated.

gastrocolocutaneous fistula: A rare iatrogenic complication of PEG tube placement in which a communication forms between the skin, transverse colon, and stomach. It occurs when a loop of transverse colon lies anteriorly to the stomach during insertion of the PEG tube and the tube is inserted through the colon unintentionally on its way into the stomach. The diagnosis is made by a gastrograffin study of the PEG tube.

gastroenterology: A subspecialty of internal medicine that primarily focuses on the evaluation and treatment of disorders of the GI tract, liver, pancreas, and biliary tract.

gastroduodenostomy: *Another term for* Billroth I.

gastroesophageal junction: The transition point between the end of the esophagus and the start of the gastric cardia. Endoscopically, it is recognized as the squamocolumnar junction (*also called* Z-line). This area is susceptible to mucosal damage from acid reflux and is the most common site to see Barrett's esophagus form.

gastroesophageal reflux disease (GERD): A disorder characterized by retrosternal burning, regurgitation, or chest pain that is primarily caused by transient relaxation of the lower esophageal sphincter, which allows gastric contents to ascend into the esophagus. It can predispose individuals to esophagitis, Barrett's esophagus, and esophageal adenocarcinoma. Treatment includes proton pump inhibitors, histamine receptor antagonists, dietary and lifestyle modification, and weight loss if obese; *also known as* acid reflux.

gastrointestinal foreign body: An object found within the GI tract that does not naturally belong there, usually due to unintentional or intentional ingestion. It often requires endoscopic or surgical extraction if unable to pass safely through the GI tract on its own.

gastrointestinal stromal tumor: A mesenchymal tumor of the GI tract, usually arising from the muscularis propria and most often found in the stomach. Immunohistochemistry tests are positive for c-kit in more than 70% of patients. Surgical resection may be necessary if associated with GI bleeding, gastric outlet obstruction, or large size.

gastrojejunostomy: A surgical connection between the stomach and jejunum; *see also* Billroth I and Billroth II.

gastroparesis: A condition of delayed gastric emptying that is not due to a true obstruction in the stomach or small intestine. It is commonly due to diabetes mellitus but is idiopathic in many cases. It is diagnosed using a gastric emptying test. Treatment includes dietary modification, frequent small meals, and pro-motility agents. In severe cases, pyloric botox injections or gastric pacemaker insertion may be indicated.

G cell: Cells found within the antrum and pylorus of the stomach whose primary function is to secrete gastrin.

genotype: Specialized genetic information or specific alleles of an individual or an individual virus. It is an important piece of information in determining treatment options for hepatitis C and, less commonly, hepatitis B. For example, different genotypes of hepatitis C respond differently to different types and duration of treatments.

giant cell hepatitis: A rare form of liver inflammation character-ized by a transformation of hepatocytes into multinucleated giant cells. There are unknown pathophysiology or triggers, and different types have been described, including neonatal, postinfantile, syncytial (in combination with autoimmune hemolytic anemia), and adult. Corticosteroids are the mainstay of treatment in the adult form.

Giardia lamblia: A protozoan parasite common in the United States and around the world that can infect the small bowel by adhering to the epithelium. Humans acquire the infection by ingesting water or food contaminated with feces, often when ingesting untreated mountain stream, lake, or well water. Clinical presentation can vary from a self-limited diarrheal illness to persistent diarrhea with weight loss. It can cause chronic diarrhea in an immunocompromised host but is usually treated effectively by metronidazole.

Gilbert's syndrome: A common genetic disorder of reduced activity of a bilirubin conjugation enzyme—UDP glucuronyltransferase—resulting in benign unconjugated hyperbilirubinemia. During periods of fasting or sickness or while taking certain drugs, levels of unconjugated bilirubin may increase further and cause mild jaundice.

globulin gap: The numerical difference between total protein and albumin on a hepatic laboratory panel. It is calculated by subtracting the albumin concentration from the total protein concentration. If elevated (more than 4 g/dL), it suggests the presence of an alternative protein in the blood, such as paraproteins in myeloma or immunoglobulins in autoimmune hepatitis. In addition, viral hepatitis often has an increased globulin gap.

globus: The sensation of feeling a lump or tightness in the throat.

glomus tumor: An uncommon, malignant vascular tumor derived from a glomulus, a group of vessels that link arterioles to venules. Typically, it is found on the skin of the extremities but infrequently can be found in the mucosa of the GI tract.

glucagonoma: An endocrine tumor of the pancreas that secretes glucagon. The clinical presentation includes migratory necrolytic erythema (specific type of dermatitis), new onset diabetes mellitus, and weight loss. It can be benign, but the majority of cases are malignant, with metastases present at the time of diagnosis.

glutamine: An important amino acid that functions as the main source of energy for the enterocytes (intestinal cells).

glutaraldehyde-induced proctocolitis: A chemical colitis induced as a result of inadequate rinsing of a colonoscope after the disinfectant chemical, glutaraldehyde, is applied. It presents as abdominal pain, bloody diarrhea, or tenesmus 48 to 72 hours after a colonoscopy.

gluten: A storage protein found in certain grains, including wheat, rye, and barley, that is the causative agent of celiac disease.

gluten free: A US Food and Drug Administration-proposed label used on manufactured foods that contain less than 20 parts per million of gluten.

gluten-free diet: Removing all sources of gluten from the diet, such as wheat, rye, barley, and any gluten-containing manufactured foods or products. This diet is used for for patients with celiac disease, gluten intolerance, and gluten-sensitive enteropathy.

gluten intolerance: A term used to describe chronic diarrhea and abdominal pain syndromes that respond to gluten-free diet but do not meet the criteria for diagnosis of celiac disease.

gluten-sensitive enteropathy: *Another term for* celiac disease or celiac sprue, although it may also be used to describe symptoms consistent with celiac disease in the absence of traditional serologic markers or histologic findings that would otherwise signify the presence of celiac disease.

glycogen acanthosis: A benign endoscopic and histologic finding of the esophagus seen as areas of epidermal thickening due to excess glycogen deposition. Severe presentation of this condition is associated with Cowden's disease.

gold probe: A multipolar electrocautery device typically used through an endoscope in the treatment of GI bleeding.

Gorlin syndrome: An autosomal dominant disorder that results in a wide spectrum of defects including early onset basal cell carcinoma, central nervous system defects, and gastric hamartomatous polyps; also known as *basal cell nevus syndrome* or *nevoid basal cell carcinoma syndrome.*

graft-versus-host disease (GVHD): A major source of morbidity and mortality seen in transplant recipients in whom donor T-cells recognize host alloantigens, resulting in proliferation and differentiation of effector cells that are activated against host cells. The result is tissue injury in any part of the body, most commonly noted in the skin, GI tract, and liver.

granulomatous gastritis: Inflammation of the stomach characterized by the formation of granulomas, which are collections of activated macrophages that become epithelioid in appearance. It can be associated with Crohn's disease, sarcoidosis, Whipple's disease, and other rare conditions. This condition may be responsive to corticosteroid treatment.

granulomatous hepatitis: Inflammation of the liver characterized by the formation of granulomas, which are collections of activated macrophages that become epithelioid in appearance. Most commonly, it is caused by sarcoidosis, tuberculosis, or a drug reaction and is diagnosed by liver biopsy.

ground glass hepatocytes: A histologic finding on liver biopsy in which liver parenchymal cells have an eosinophilic, finely granular cytoplasm. This finding is most often associated with chronic active hepatitis B infection or, less likely, a drug reaction.

guaiac test: A stool-based test of poor accuracy used for CRC screening. A positive test suggests microscopic blood loss from the GI tract, which may be associated with an undiagnosed malignancy or polyp.

gynecomastia: Enlargement of male breast tissue. It can occur as a part of normal development at certain stages of male life, be pathologic due to excess estrogen (eg, cirrhosis), or be a side effect of a medication (eg, spironolactone).

H2-blocker: A class of medications used in the treatment of peptic ulcer disease and GERD. H2-blockers target the histamine receptor H2 in gastric parietal cells, leading to decreased gastric acid production. Medications in this class include cimetidine, famotidine, and ranitidine.

halitosis: *Another term for* bad breath, which may be a symptom associated with a Zenker's diverticulum, GERD, or gastroparesis.

HALO ablation: *See* BARRX ablation.

hamartoma: A benign mass composed of mature cells in which the cells replicate at the same rate as the surrounding tissue. These rare tumors can occur anywhere in the GI tract but most often affect the colon and small bowel and are commonly seen in familial polyposis syndromes. They are most often single, pedunculated, and found in the rectosigmoid. They may cause obstructive symptoms when large.

hazard ratio: A statistic used in survival data to describe how often a particular event happens in one group versus another over the same time period.

heartburn: A sensation of burning pain located behind the breastbone often radiating toward the neck. The term is often used interchangeably with GERD, acid reflux, and dyspepsia.

Helicobacter heilmanii: *A* gram-negative helical bacteria previously known as *Gastrospirillum hominis*. Most commonly affects cats, dogs, and primates but is implicated in up to 6% of human gastric infections. Most commonly, it can cause chronic gastritis, but it may also cause peptic ulcer disease (duodenal more commonly than gastric) and has been rarely associated with gastric carcinoma and mucosa-associated lymphoid tissue.

Fenkel JM, ed.
Quick Reference Dictionary for GI and Hepatology (pp 84-99).
© 2014 Taylor & Francis Group.

Helicobacter pylori: A gram-negative, spiral shaped, microaerophilic bacteria that infects approximately two-thirds of all people in the world. It is spread through contaminated food and water or via mouth-to-mouth transmission. It is implicated in the formation of peptic ulcer disease, gastric adenocarcinoma, and gastric mucosa-associated lymphoid tissue (MALT) lymphoma. Endoscopic biopsy, serologic testing, or stool antigen testing can be used for diagnosis. Treatment involves a combination of taking at least two antibiotics and the use of a proton pump inhibitor for 10 to 14 days.

Heller myotomy: A surgical procedure developed for the treatment of achalasia that can be performed open or laparoscopically. It entails the division of the hypertrophied gastroesophageal junction mucosa in a direction longitudinal to the mucosa, extending from the proximal aspect of the hypertrophied muscle and approximately 2 cm onto the stomach. The procedure is often performed with a fundoplication to prevent GERD postoperatively.

hemangioendothelioma: *See* epitheliod hemangioendothelioma.

hemangiomatosis: The presence of multiple hemangiomas in one organ, most often the liver, that can cause biliary obstruction, depending on the location of the lesions, or portal hypertension if a critical mass of liver parenchyma is replaced by hemangiomas. It has been associated with recurrent acute cholangitis and portal hypertensive-related bleeding in advanced cases, and liver transplantation can be considered in these situations.

hematemesis: The act of vomiting red or dark coffee ground–appearing blood in the setting of acute upper GI hemorrhage. Common causes include variceal hemorrhage, peptic ulcer disease, and erosive esophagitis. Endoscopy is the first diagnostic and therapeutic step after acute stabilization and volume resuscitation.

hematochezia: The passage of bright red or maroon-colored blood from the rectum usually mixed with stool, indicating a lower GI source of bleeding or brisk upper GI bleed. It is most commonly due to diverticulosis or hemorrhoids, although angioectasisas, IBD, colon cancer, and foregut variceal bleeding may also present with hematochezia.

hematoxylin and eosin (H&E) stain: A common histologic technique using H&E staining. Hemotoxylin is a basic dye that stains acidic (or basophilic) structures blue or purple. These structures include DNA in the nucleus and RNA in ribosomes and rough endoplasmic reticulum. Eosin is an acidic dye that stains basic (or acidophilic) structures pink. These structures include cytoplasm and intracellular membranes.

hemobilia: Hemorrhage into the biliary tract that most commonly presents as upper GI bleeding (melena or hematemesis) but can also present as jaundice or right upper quadrant pain. Causes include liver trauma, vasculitis, vascular malformations, complications of biliary procedures, and hepatic tumors.

hemochromatosis: An autosomal recessive inherited disease that results from excessive iron deposition in cells of the body, particularly the liver. It is most commonly due to a mutation in the HFE gene (C282Y or H63D). The body absorbs excess dietary iron and is unable to properly excrete it, resulting in organ dysfunction. The most common clinical manifestations are cirrhosis, diabetes mellitus, hypogonadism, arthritis, hepatocellular carcinoma, and cardiomyopathy. Treatment before end-organ dysfunction is primarily with phlebotomy, but iron chelators may also be used. Liver transplantation is curative, but is usually only pursued if end-stage liver disease or hepatocellular carcinoma occurs.

hemolysis, elevated liver enzymes, and low platelet count (HELLP) syndrome: A pregnancy-related condition occurring most often in the 3rd trimester that can be life threatening for both the baby and the mother. Jaundice, thrombocytopenia, anemia, edema, abdominal pain, nausea/vomiting, and elevated lactate dehydrogenase are common signs/symptoms of the condition. Urgent delivery is the treatment of choice; *compare* acute fatty liver of pregnancy; *see* Appendix 8.

hemoperitoneum: The presence of blood in the peritoneal cavity that occurs spontaneously (eg, from rupture of a hepatic adenoma or hepatocellular cancer) or iatrogenically (eg, as a complication of paracentesis or abdominal surgery). In addition to supportive care, surgical consultation is often needed.

hemorrhoids: Normally occurring vascular cushions in the anal canal that aid stool continence but can become swollen or inflamed, leading to anorectal discomfort and bleeding. Common causes include obesity, pregnancy, a low-fiber diet, and constipation. They can be characterized as external if they are located below the dentate line and arise from the inferior hemorrhoidal veins or internal if they are found above the dentate line and arise from rectal veins.

hemosiderin: Intracellular, iron-containing protein complex that is produced by the phagocytic digestion of hemoglobin. It can be visualized in cells or found in urine. Its presence in urine usually suggests recent blood transfusion or active hemolysis.

hemosiderosis: Abnormal accumulation of the iron-storage product hemosiderin within tissues (particularly the liver and spleen), most often in the setting of a patient with end-stage renal disease who is undergoing hemodialysis or a patient with a chronic anemia condition requiring multiple transfusions.

Henoch-Schönlein purpura (HSP): An autoimmune, IgA-mediated vasculitis that is most commonly a result of immune complex deposition after infection with Group A *Streptococcus,* mycoplasma, Epstein-Barr virus, or varicella. It usually presents with palpable dark red lesions called *purpura* on the lower extremities, abdominal pain, joint pains, or renal involvement. The abdominal pain found in Henoch-Schönlein purpura can be associated with vomiting and be colicky in nature. Rarely, hematemesis, intussusception, bowel infarction, or hepato-splenomegaly occur.

hepatectomy: Surgical removal of a portion of the liver, typically for the excision of a mass lesion, or the entire liver in the setting of liver transplantation. The procedure can be performed open, laparascopically, or using robotic assistance, depending on the location of the mass and patient factors.

hepatic: Of or pertaining to the liver.

hepatic adenoma: A benign, solid neoplasm typically seen in women aged 20 to 40 years that is often induced by estrogen exposure from oral contraceptives. When larger than 5 cm in size, surgical resection is recommended because there is a significant risk of spontaneous rupture leading to intraperitoneal hemorrhage, as well as a potential small risk of malignant transformation. If smaller than 5 cm, observation and surveillance of estrogen-containing compounds can be an option. Diagnosis is made with imaging, and biopsy can be performed if the radiologic diagnosis is uncertain.

hepatic artery: A branch of the celiac artery that supplies oxygenated blood to the pancreas, duodenum, pylorus, liver, and bile ducts. The liver is supplied by a branch called the proper hepatic artery, a component of the portal triad that further bifurcates into the right and left hepatic arteries. Ischemic injury to the hepatic artery can lead to biliary damage because the bile ducts receive their entire nutritional blood flow through it, whereas the liver is less susceptible due to dual blood supply from the hepatic artery and portal vein; *also referred to as* the common hepatic artery.

hepatic cyst: A benign, thin-walled, fluid-filled lesion found within the liver. It can be solitary or there could be multiple, particularly in association with polycystic kidney disease. Treatment is not typically required unless the cyst is large and extends into the capsule of the liver causing pain or compresses the inferior vena cava causing lower extremity edema. If treatment is necessary, options include percutaneous drainage, percutaneous alcohol injection, and surgical marsupialization (unroofing).

hepatic encephalopathy: Alteration in the level of consciousness and mental acuity as a result of acute or chronic liver failure leading to decreased clearance of ammonia and other toxic metabolites. It is graded by the West Haven criteria, and a formal diagnosis can be made with neuropsychiatric testing, although clinical impression in the right patient is usually sufficient. Early symptoms can include day/night reversal, confusion, irritability, and forgetfulness. More advanced symptoms include stupor and coma. Treatment options include the prescription of lactulose or rifaximin and the management of potential triggers, including infection, bleeding, medication nonadherence, or hepatocellular carcinoma.

hepatic flexure: The section of colon located at the junction of the ascending and transverse colons that in situ is typically near the liver. A bluish submucosal hue can be seen in the colon during colonoscopy at the location.

hepatic hemangioma: A benign liver lesion, also known as a cavernous hemangioma, that is composed of dilated blood vessels. Hepatic hemangiomas occur more commonly in women and are usually diagnosed between the ages of 30 and 50 years. These lesions are rarely symptomatic and are usually discovered incidentally on imaging performed for other reasons. No specific treatment is necessary unless the hemangioma is so large that it causes pain or bleeding. Diagnosis is made with cross-sectional imaging, and biopsies are generally not recommended due to the intense vascularity of the lesion.

hepatic hydrothorax: A pleural effusion that occurs in less than 10% of patients with cirrhosis and end-stage liver disease, usually on the right side, but can occur on the left or bilaterally in less than 5% of patients. Diuretic therapy is the first-line therapy, but thoracentesis may be used for patients with acute shortness of breath or those intolerant to diuretics. If thoracentesis needs to be performed more than once per week, a TIPS procedure is indicated, as is a liver transplant evaluation.

hepaticojejunostomy: A surgical anastomosis of the hepatic duct to the jejunum, typically performed to treat benign or malignant strictures of the biliary tree or as part of a liver transplant operation for biliary reconstruction in a patient with primary sclerosing cholangitis or prior biliary tract surgery.

hepatic venous pressure gradient (HVPG): An indirect measurement of portal pressure calculated by subtracting the wedged hepatic venous pressure from the free hepatic venous pressure during a transvenous pressure study. An HVPG score between 1 and 5 is normal; greater than 5 is considered portal hypertension; and greater than 10 is clinically significant portal hypertension (ie, the pressure above which ascites and variceal hemorrhage are more likely to occur).

hepatitis A: An RNA virus transmitted via fecal-oral transmission that causes acute inflammation of the liver. Most patients infected with hepatitis A are asymptomatic, but the likelihood of developing symptoms increases with age and 0.5% of those infected can develop fulminant liver failure. Acute infection is diagnosed by the presence of hepatitis A IgM approximately 2 weeks after being infected. Resolution of infection leads to the formation of hepatitis A IgG, which confers immunity to reinfection. IgG is also present after vaccination, and it is recommended that patients with chronic liver disease, including those with chronic infection with hepatitis B or C, are vaccinated.

hepatitis B: A partially double-stranded DNA hepadnavirus that can lead to acute or chronic hepatitis. Infection is spread through bodily fluids, with the exception of breast milk. Viral infection is endemic in most developing nations, where infection is typically due to perinatal transmission. Acute infection tends to be self-limited and can be asymptomatic, but rarely it can cause acute liver failure. Hepatitis B infection is cleared more frequently the older the patient is at the time of infection. Infection can also be chronic and lead to cirrhosis or hepatocellular carcinoma. Treatment is with anti-viral medications; *see* Appendix 11.

hepatitis C: An RNA virus belonging to the flaviviridae family that was known as non-A non-B hepatitis until 1989. It is spread through blood contamination; this primarily refers to injection drug use, blood transfusions, military blood exposure, and tattoos but can also refer to less common methods of acquisition, such as intranasal drug use, contaminated personal care items, dialysis, or high-risk sexual contact. Acute infection is often asymptomatic, and 10% to 20% of people clear infection spontaneously. Chronic infection occurs in more than 80% of patients, and 20% to 50% will develop cirrhosis over a period of 20 to 30 years. Hepatitis C is also a major risk factor for hepatocellular carcinoma. Six main genotypes (numbered 1 to 6) exist. Treatment has traditionally included interferon injections in combination with oral ribavirin. Since 2011, several new direct-acting antiviral agents have been introduced in the marketplace, and the management of hepatitis C is expected to change dramatically over the next 3 to 5 years; *see* Appendix 4.

hepatitis D: A small, defective RNA virus that requires hepatitis B viral infection to infect hepatocytes. When coinfection occurs, patients are more likely to experience acute liver failure. With superinfection, hepatitis D hastens the progression to cirrhosis. Like hepatitis B, the hepatitis D virus is spread through bodily fluids. The underlying hepatitis B infection should be treated to cure the hepatitis D.

hepatitis E: An RNA virus that can cause acute hepatitis through fecal-oral transmission. Disease is usually self-limited and is fatal in less than 2% of patients. When infection occurs in pregnancy, it is more commonly associated with fulminant hepatic failure, most notably when infection occurs in the third trimester. It is also being recognized as a potential source of chronic hepatitis in patients who are immunocompromised, particularly those who have undergone solid organ transplants. Treatment is supportive for acute hepatitis E, but ribavirin may be helpful in the chronic form. Diagnosis is made by measuring hepatitis E IgM/G or quantitative RNA viral load. These tests are not widely available and may require confirmation by the Center for Disease Control.

hepatitis G: An RNA virus also known as GB virus C that is a member of the flaviviridae family. It is spread through sexual contact, blood, and vertical transmission. The carrier rate is 2% to 5% in the general population, including 1% to 1.5% of blood donors in the United States. Unlike other hepatitis viruses, hepatitis G is not believed to cause liver disease. It is commonly transmitted with hepatitis B and C and HIV infection, and it is thought to possibly slow the progression of HIV infection.

hepatobiliary scintigraphy: A radionuclide study using Technetium-99m that is performed for functional assessment of the hepatobiliary system or integrity of the hepatobiliary tree; *also known as* a HIDA scan. A qualitative examination can be used in the diagnosis of acute cholecystitis, and a quantitative examination with gallbladder stimulation by cholecystokinin evaluates gallbladder function to diagnose gallbladder dyskinesia or chronic cholecystitis.

hepatocellular carcinoma: A primary cancer of the liver that arises from hepatocytes and is one of the top ten most common cancers worldwide. It can be diagnosed by gadolinium-enhanced MRI, contrast-enhanced CT, or directed liver biopsy. Risk factors include chronic hepatitis B or C infection, cirrhosis, hemochromatosis, exposure to aflatoxin, iron overload, and chronic alcohol abuse. It is often asymptomatic at diagnosis and detected by screening but may present as abdominal pain, easy bruising, jaundice, hemoperitoneum, or newly decompensated cirrhosis. Treatment options include locoregional therapy with chemoembolization or radioembolization, surgical resection, liver transplantation, oral or intravenous chemotherapy, or palliative care depending on the underlying liver function and stage at which the cancer is diagnosed.

hepatocellular jaundice: Yellowing of the skin and mucous membranes as a result of the accumulation of bilirubin in the blood secondary to liver cell injury. Etiologies include acute or chronic hepatitis, decompensated cirrhosis, metabolic derangement, or hepatotoxicity from medications, dietary supplements, or alcohol.

hepatocyte: The primary functional cell of the liver composing approximately 80% of the liver mass. Its primary roles are protein synthesis and storage, drug metabolism, gluconeogenesis, and cholesterol formation.

hepatolenticular degeneration: *Another term for* Wilson's disease.

hepatology: A subspecialty of internal medicine that focuses on the study of liver disease.

hepatomegaly: The presence of an enlarged liver on physical examination or imaging. It may be a manifestation of an acute injury from drug toxicity or viral hepatitis or may be chronically enlarged in patients who abuse alcohol, have metabolic or storage disorders, or have infiltrative disorders, such as lymphoma or sarcoidosis.

hepatopancreatic ampulla: *Another term for* ampulla of Vater.

hepatopulmonary syndrome: A serious complication of portal hypertension and end-stage liver disease diagnosed by the presence of hypoxemia and transpulmonic shunting due to pulmonary vascular dilation. Patients with this condition receive extra priority on the liver transplant wait list, but if hypoxemia is significant, performing a transplant may not be safe. Patients may complain of increased shortness of breath while sitting upright (platypnea) and have lower blood oxygenation measured by pulse oximetry or arterial blood gas while sitting upright (orthodeoxia).

hepatorenal syndrome: A decline in renal function as a result of cirrhosis and portal hypertension. It is believed to occur as a result of splanchnic vasodilation causing compensatory vasoconstriction of the renal circulation, resulting in worsening renal function. There are two types of hepatorenal syndrome. Type 1 is rapidly progressive, results in a doubling of the serum creatinine within 2 weeks, and usually occurs in patients with spontaneous bacterial peritonitis or acute GI bleeding. Type 2 progresses slowly over weeks to months and most commonly occurs in patients with refractory ascites. Hepatorenal syndrome is a diagnosis of exclusion and is characterized by a urine sodium level less than 10 μmol/L and lack of response to a fluid challenge with intravenous albumin or saline. Treatment includes octreotide injections, midodrine, albumin infusions, and rapid liver transplant evaluation.

hepatosplenic T-cell lymphoma: A rare malignancy with a poor prognosis that comprises approximately 1% of all lymphomas in which malignant CD3 positive T cells occupy space in the hepatic or splenic sinusoids. It may present as new onset ascites, jaundice, or as abdominal pain with fevers, chills, and weight loss. It can be a rare side effect of immunomodulator and biologic therapy, particularly when used in combination in young men being treated for IBD.

hepatosplenomegaly: Simultaneous enlargement of both the liver and spleen on physical examination or imaging. It is most commonly found in infectious mononucleosis, acute viral hepatitis, portal hypertension from hepatic venous outflow obstruction, alcoholic liver disease, or lysosomal storage diseases.

hepatotoxicity: Injury to the liver as a result of a chemical, substance, medication, or herbal supplement. Both predictable (acetaminophen) and unpredictable hepatotoxicity can occur. Most instances of hepatotoxicity are self-limited, and treatment is supportive with withdrawal of the offending agent. Rarely, hepatotoxicity can progress to fulminant liver failure, requiring urgent transplantation.

hereditary angioedema: An autosomal dominant disorder that usually presents in the second to fourth decades of life with intermittent swelling of mucosal or cutaneous surfaces; *also known as* Quincke's disease. It is due to a deficiency in C1 esterase inhibitor and can cause bowel wall edema, presenting as nausea and vomiting. Genetic mutations in the SERPING1 or F12 gene are responsible for the disease.

hereditary nonpolyposis colon cancer (HNPCC): An autosomal dominant disorder that results in impaired DNA mismatch repair. Affected patients have an approximate 80% lifetime risk of developing CRC, as well as an increased risk of developing endometrial, skin, brain, ovarian, gastric, hepatobiliary, and genitourinary malignancies; *another term for* Lynch syndrome.

hereditary pancreatitis: An autosomal dominant condition with incomplete penetrance that causes chronic pancreatitis. The disease usually manifests before age 10 years with abdominal pain and acute pancreatitis resulting in pancreatic calcification. Gradual decline in pancreatic exocrine and endocrine function later ensue. This condition also carries an increased risk of pancreatic cancer. Most cases are caused by a mutation in the PRSS1 gene.

hernia: Protrusion of an organ or fascia through a weakened area in the muscular wall that normally contains it. Common sites for GI-related herniation include the diaphragmatic hiatus, the umbilicus, and the inguinal area.

herpes simplex esophagitis: Infection of the esophagus by herpes simplex virus resulting in inflammation, odynophagia, dysphagia, and the risk of GI bleeding. It is more common in patients who are immunosuppressed but can occur in those who are immunocompetent. Diagnosis is made with endoscopic biopsies, and treatment is with herpes-specific antiviral therapy.

Heyde's syndrome: A clinical correlation between aortic stenosis and angiodysplasia of the GI tract leading to GI bleeding. The aortic stenosis is thought to cause an acquired form of von Willebrand disease, increasing the risk of bleeding. It is named for Dr. Edward Heyde, who first described this connection in 1958.

HFE gene: Located on chromosome 6, this genetic material encodes a protein that regulates iron absorption. Mutations (with the C282Y gene being the most common) result in hemochromatosis. Commercial testing for this mutation is available in most laboratories.

hiatal hernia: Protrusion of the proximal stomach into the mediastinum through the esophageal hiatus. Sliding hiatal hernias occur when the proximal stomach and gastroesophageal junction herniate toward the head through the esophageal diaphragmatic hiatus and comprise 95% of cases. Sliding hernias may increase GERD. Paraesophageal hernias are more rare, occurring when the stomach and esophagus stay in their anatomic position but a section of stomach herniates alongside the normal anatomy in the hiatus, putting the patient at risk for strangulation. This type of hernia may require surgical correction.

Hirschsprung's disease: An embryologic defect leading to an aganglionic colon due to the failure of neural crest cells to migrate during gestation, most commonly affecting the rectosigmoid or rectum alone. Clinically, it results in failure of the colon to relax in front of a progressing food bolus, causing abdominal distention, constipation, vomiting, and the hesitancy to feed. It is more common in boys and is often noticed within the first few days of life when meconium is not passed as expected. Children with Down syndrome have an increased risk of this condition. Anorectal manometry can confirm the diagnosis, and surgical correction is needed.

histamine: An organic compound synthesized within the body's mast cells, basophils, and gastric enterochromaffin-like cells whose primarily roles include stimulating gastric acid secretion and triggering immune and inflammatory responses.

histoplasmosis: A type of fungal infection due to *Histoplasma capsulatum,* an endemic mycosis in the Ohio and Mississippi River valleys. The fungus is carried in bird and bat droppings, and infection occurs through the inhalation of microconidia when the soil is disrupted. The microconidia are engulfed by phagocytes in humans and then begin to bud, with the infection spreading through the lymphatic system. In individuals who are immunocompetent, infection may be subclinical or cause a respiratory infection. In individuals who are immunosuppressed, disease is often disseminated and has a poor prognosis. Diagnosis is made with biopsy and culture of the affected organ.

HLA B27: A specific type of HLA highly associated with ankylosing spondylitis. It is also associated with the development of reactive arthritis after infection with an enteric organism, such as *Campylobacter jejuni.*

HLA DQ2/DQ8: A specific type of HLA highly associated with a genetic predisposition for the development of celiac disease. DQ2 is seen in approximately 30% of the White population and is positive in approximately 95% of individuals with celiac disease. DQ8 also predisposes individuals to developing celiac disease but has a lower prevalence than DQ2.

hot biopsy: A type of forceps endoscopic biopsy taken with a high-frequency coagulation current to aid in the eradication of remnant polyp tissue. It is most often used to remove small sessile or pedunculated polyps and occasionally for larger, sessile polyps. Its use is less frequent now than in the past due to concerns about more residual polyps than with cold biopsy or snare cautery polypectomy, as well as increased risk of postpolypectomy bleeding and perforation when used in the right colon.

human epidermal growth factor 2 (HER2/neu): A receptor tyrosine kinase that is encoded by the ErbB2 gene, whose overexpression has been linked to more aggressive forms of breast, uterine, ovarian, and gastric cancers.

human immunodeficiency virus (HIV): A lentivirus transmitted through bodily fluids that infects cells in the immune system. HIV causes destruction of CD4+ cells and can evolve into AIDS. It can cause many abnormalities in the GI tract; *see* Appendix 18.

human leukocyte antigens (HLA): A class of genes that are the human equivalent of the major histocompatibility complex. HLAs are involved in immune function, including the complement system and the presentation of antigens to lymphocytes.

human papillomavirus (HPV): A virus within the papillomavirus genus that infects the epithelial cells of mucous membranes and skin. Infection may be asymptomatic or can result in genital or anal warts, cervical cancer, and possibly an increased risk of esophageal cancer. The HPV-6 type is most commonly associated with anal warts.

hydrochloric acid: The main component of gastric secretions that acidifies the stomach, aiding in the digestive process by enzymatic activation and sterilization of food. Its production is inhibited by proton pump inhibitors.

hydroxyiminodiacetic acid (HIDA) scan: A nuclear medicine test used to diagnose gallbladder, biliary tree, or liver abnormalities. A radioactive tracer is injected through an IV and traces the flow of bile in the body. HIDA stands for hydroxyiminodiacetic acid, the original tracer used in the test. Both qualitative (to diagnose acute cholecystitis or bile leak) and quantitative (to diagnose chronic cholecystitis) HIDA scans can be performed.

hyperbilirubinemia: Elevated bilirubin concentration in the blood. This condition can result from biliary obstruction, genetic errors in bilirubin metabolism, medications, sepsis, infection, or acute or chronic liver disease. Treatment is targeted at the specific etiology. Levels above 3 mg/dL usually result in visible scleral icterus and skin jaundice.

hypercalcemia: An elevated calcium level in the blood that may occur as a result of bone breakdown, chronic granulomatous disease, or malignancy.

hyperechoic lesion: An ultrasonographic finding that appears brighter in intensity due to the increased amplitude of the returned ultrasonic waves. Bone and dense tissue are most commonly hyperechoic. Malignant lesions are more commonly hypoechoic, whereas benign findings, such as hemangiomas, are more commonly hyperechoic. However, neuroendocrine tumors may present as hyperechoic lesions, thus the finding warrants additional cross-sectional imaging and a more detailed evaluation.

hypergastrinemia: Elevated blood levels of gastrin that can be seen in Zollinger-Ellison syndrome or autoimmune gastritis. Chronic use of proton pump inhibitors can also cause increased gastrin levels, although not usually as high as in patients with Zollinger-Ellison syndrome.

hyperplastic polyp: The most common type of nonmalignant polyp found in the colon. They are composed of normal colonic cells and are typically difficult to differentiate from adenomatous polyps on visual inspection. Usually, they are smaller than 5 mm and are more commonly located in the rectosigmoid portion of the colon. They are not considered malignant; however, lesions larger than 2 cm have a small risk of malignant transformation.

hyperplastic polyposis syndrome: A rare colorectal polyp syndrome defined by (1) at least 5 hyperplastic polyps proximal to the sigmoid colon with at least 2 larger than 1 cm, (2) hyperplastic polyps found in a patient with a first-degree relative who has hyperplastic polyposis, and (3) more than 30 hyperplastic polyps throughout the colon. Polyps are typically flat and large, and the syndrome increases the lifetime risk of colon cancer. Although an inherited disorder, no mutation has been identified currently.

hypertriglyceridemia: Elevated levels of triglycerides in the blood that can be acquired or inherited. Consistently elevated triglycerides can predispose patients to the formation of xanthomas, retinal deposits, heart disease, or pancreatitis.

hypertrophied anal papilla: Thickened squamous epithelium that originates from squamous epithelium below the dentate line often detected on a retroflexion maneuver in the rectum during colonoscopy. It appears as a whitish-colored, slightly raised area that is firm on palpation. It typically has no symptoms but can be mistaken for a polyp and sampled accidentally during a procedure. It may occur more commonly in patients with chronic fissures.

hypoechoic lesion: An ultrasonographic finding that appears darker in intensity, implying a more solid nature to the mass. It is often concerning for malignancy. In the liver, hypoechoic lesions are worrisome for hepatocellular carcinoma or metastatic cancer. Less commonly, focal nodular hyperplasia or hemangiomas can appear as hypoechoic lesions. Cross-sectional imaging is the next step to evaluate a hypoechoic lesion.

icterus/icteric: Yellowing of the eyes, skin, or mucous membranes as a result of hyperbilirubinemia.

idiopathic gastroparesis: Chronic delayed gastric emptying without a readily identifiable cause. This type of gastroparesis accounts for up to half of all cases and is often thought to be the result of an autoimmune phenomenon after viral infection or due to psychiatric illness. Treatment is the same as any other type of gastroparesis.

interleukin-2 (IL-2) inhibitor: Antagonist of IL-2, a key cytokine in T cell–mediate immunity, mainly used in the prevention or treatment of acute cellular rejection in solid organ transplantation. Medications in this class include basiliximab and dacluzimab. IL-2 can be directly inhibited by the agents basiliximab and dacluzimab. IL-2 production can also be inhibited by corticosteroids and calcineurin inhibitors.

IL28B: A gene located on chromosome 19 that is thought to encode a cytokine activated during viral infection. A single nucleotide polymorphism located near the IL28B gene helps predict responsiveness to interferon-based hepatitis C treatment. A TT genotype portends a poor response to treatment, whereas the CC genotype predicts a higher cure rate and potentially shorter treatment duration. A mixed TC genotype predicts intermediate responsiveness.

ileal conduit: A surgical procedure in which a loop of ileum is used as a reservoir for urine after the bladder is removed. The ureters are diverted into a section of ileum that is detached from the bowel and connected to the abdominal wall via a stoma, through which urine is collected. It is most commonly performed for patients with bladder cancer requiring cystectomy.

Fenkel JM, ed.
Quick Reference Dictionary for GI and Hepatology (pp 100-108).
© 2014 Taylor & Francis Group.

ileoanal pouch: A surgically created reservoir formed by the connection of the ileum to the anus located in the position formerly occupied by the rectum in patients who have their colon removed for refractory colitis, those with recurrent symptomatic diverticular disease, or those with colon cancer or for the prevention of colon cancer in inherited cancer syndromes. The pouch, *also known as* a J-pouch, serves as a reservoir for stool, which can then be evacuated through the anus.

ileocecal valve: A physiologic muscle sphincter located at the junction of the ileum and colon that is a common site of inflammation in patients with IBD. It is also one of the landmarks in performing a colonoscopy, and photographic evidence of reaching the area is a quality indicator.

ileocecectomy: The surgical excision of the terminal ileum (the most distal part of the small intestine) and cecum often performed for patients with Crohn's disease. It can also be performed for right-sided colon cancers, appendiceal carcinoid tumors larger than 2 cm at the greatest dimension, complicated right-sided diverticulitis, or other diseases confined to the distal small bowel or proximal colon.

ileostomy: The surgical procedure used to create an opening into the ileum from the skin by creating a stoma. It can be created temporarily in the management of perforated diverticulitis or large bowel obstruction or be permanent in someone with a total proctocolectomy.

ileum: The last and longest section of the small intestine that connects to the cecum. It is responsible for the absorption of vitamin B_{12} and bile salts and for the final steps in the digestion and absorption of protein and carbohydrates. It is also the most common site in the GI tract for inflammation from Crohn's disease.

ileus: Significant hypomotility of the GI tract, particularly after surgery or general anesthesia, resembling a bowel obstruction without evidence of mechanical obstruction. Symptoms include abdominal distention/bloating, pain, nausea, vomiting, and constipation. Treatment is bowel rest, nasogastric tube decompression, intravenous hydration, and avoidance of medications than can further slow gut motility.

immunoglobulin: A type of glycoprotein antibody whose function is to participate in the immune response. In humans, each immunoglobulin is composed of two heavy chains and two light polypeptide chains. Each chain has a constant and a variable region. Variable regions are responsible for antigen binding, whereas constant regions of the heavy chain are responsible for activating various immune functions. Many types of immunoglobulins exist and have more specific roles in the immune response.

immunoglobulin A (IgA): The main immunoglobulin in bodily secretions, including saliva, tears, and respiratory and GI secretions. It helps prevent adherence of microorganisms to mucous membranes. Patients with IgA deficiency are more prone to GI and respiratory infections. Deposition of IgA in the kidneys can cause a chronic kidney disease called IgA nephropathy.

immunoglobulin E (IgE): A type of antibody that prevents infection with parasites and protozoa and plays a role in hypersensitivity reactions. It is only found in mammals and does not cross the placenta. Elevated serum levels are often found in atopic patients and patients with chronic parasitic infections, particularly of the GI tract.

immunoglobulin G (IgG): A type of antibody that accounts for 80% of the circulating immunoglobulins in adults and whose major role is secondary immune response. IgG can cross the placenta, which provides passive immunity to newborns. IgG will bind antigens on pathogens to activate opsonization, complement, or direct antibody-dependent, cell-mediated cytotoxicity. Detectable IgG for a specific infection may indicate chronic or past infection.

immunoglobulin M (IgM): The predominant antibody formed during primary immunity that is expressed on B cells. IgM does not cross the placenta. It is a strong activator of complement. Detectable IgM for a specific infection indicates acute or recent infection.

immunohistochemistry: A histologic technique used in the pathology laboratory to detect antigens within a tissue sample by introducing color or fluorescent labeled antibodies directed against the desired antigen. This technique is particularly helpful in identifying the source of a metastatic malignancy.

immunomodulator: A substance that alters the normal function of the immune system. Most commonly, this refers to medications such as 6-mercaptopurine or azathioprine and is used in IBD and autoimmune hepatitis.

immunophilin: One member of a family of proteins that bind and mediate the effects of immunosuppressive agents. This class includes FK506-binding protein (target of tacrolimus) and cyclophilin (target of cyclosporine).

incisura: The anatomic location in the stomach, close to the pylorus, where there is a bend in the lesser curvature; also called the *incisura angularis*. It indicates the approximate area where the stomach begins to narrow before entering the duodenum.

India ink tattoo: A commonly used dye in endoscopic procedures to mark an abnormal area for future surveillance or surgical resection. The pigment can last for approximately 10 years. The act of marking an area with India ink is also called a chromoscopy.

infectious colitis: Inflammation of the colon as a result of infection, most often due to bacterial causes such as *C difficile, Shigella, Salmonella,* or *E coli.* Viruses (including cytomegalovirus and adenovirus) and parasitic infections *(Entamoeba histolytica)* can also cause infectious colitis. Stool cultures and colonoscopic biopsies can aid in making the diagnosis.

infectious esophagitis: Inflammation of the esophagus as a result of infection, most commonly seen in patients who are immunocompromised and usually presenting as odynophagia or dysphagia. The most common etiologies include *Candida,* Herpes simplex, HIV, and cytomegalovirus. Etiology can be determined with endoscopic biopsies.

inflammatory bowel disease (IBD): Immune-mediated chronic inflammation of the GI tract that includes the diseases Crohn's disease, ulcerative colitis, and microscopic colitis. Commonly presenting symptoms include diarrhea, abdominal pain, bloody stools, weight loss, and fevers; *see* Appendix 16.

inflammatory polyp: Lesions or growths of regenerating mucosa surrounded by areas of mucosal loss with a filiform histologic appearance. They are not malignant and are most commonly seen in the setting of IBD; *also called* inflammatory pseudopolyps.

inflammatory pseudopolyps: *Another term for* inflammatory polyp.

infrared coagulation: A type of focused energy delivered by a polymer probe tip as an ablative treatment for hemorrhoids and high-grade anal dysplasia.

inguinal: Pertaining to the lateral regions of the groin under which the inguinal canal is located. It is a common location for hernias and reactive lymphadenopathy from lower extremity infections.

inguinal hernia: Protrusion of the bowel or abdominal fascia through the inguinal canal either directly through the posterior wall of the canal or indirectly through the deep inguinal ring. Valsalva maneuvers and coughing may exacerbate a hernia. Surgery is used to correct incarcerated or symptomatic hernias, whereas small or asymptomatic ones may be observed clinically.

injection sclerotherapy: A technique in which a sclerosing agent is injected through an endoscope into a vascular lesion with the intent of treating or preventing bleeding. The most common indications for its use are bleeding esophageal or gastric varices and hemorrhoids. The sclerosant causes swelling of the blood vessel and scarring so that blood flow is diverted to collaterals. Strictures may occur as a result of injection sclerotherapy, and performing it in the esophagus also carries a small risk of mediastinitis and postprocedure chest pain.

inlet patch: A congenital malformation of ectopic gastric mucosa in the esophagus at or just proximal to the upper esophageal sphincter. These are usually asymptomatic but can increase the risk of esophagitis, webs, or strictures of the esophagus. Diagnosis is usually incidental during an upper endoscopy performed for another reason.

interface hepatitis: A histologic term used to describe inflammation located in the area between the portal track and the lobule in the liver. It is a pattern of inflammation often seen in autoimmune hepatitis and less commonly in viral hepatitis. This finding is also known as piecemeal necrosis.

interferons: Class of cytokines with antiviral, immunomodulating, and antiproliferative properties. Conditions that have been treated with interferons include warts, multiple sclerosis, hepatitis B virus, and, most commonly, hepatitis C virus.

internal anal sphincter: A thickened, circular layer of smooth muscle proximal to the external anal sphincter that is tonically contracted and provides the majority of the anal sphincter's resting tone. Its primary role is to maintain fecal continence, and it is innervated by the enteric nervous system.

intestinal ganglioneuromatosis: A rare condition defined by the presence of ganglion cells, Schwann cells, and nerve fibers in the bowel wall, most commonly affecting the ileum, colon, and appendix. It may lead to thickening of the bowel wall, polyp formation, or nodularity of the bowel wall, predisposing the bowel wall to stricture formation and mimicking Crohn's disease. This is mostly a disease diagnosed in children and may have an association with multiple endocrine neoplasia type 2B (MEN2B).

intestinal lymphangiectasia: A chronic condition of the small intestine characterized by diffusely dilated lymphatics of the intestinal mucosa that leads to protein losing enteropathy. It may be primary or secondary. The primary form is seen in childhood as a dilation of mesenteric lymphatics and is thought to be an embryonic developmental defect. The secondary form is the result of lymphatic obstruction secondary to scarring, trauma, or infection. Both forms lead to diarrhea, weight loss, growth retardation, and malabsorption of proteins and lipids. Focal areas of lymphangiectasia are often seen on wireless capsule endoscopy and have undetermined significance.

intestinal metaplasia: Transformation of gastric epithelium into instestinal-type columnar epithelium that is divided into three types. Type I is composed of fully formed small intestinal epithelium with goblet, absorptive, and Paneth cells. Types II and III are less formed than type I and have goblet cells interspersed with gastric type mucin cells. *H pylori* infection may predispose individuals to this condition in the stomach, and it is believed to be premalignant to gastric adenocarcinoma. When occurring at the gastroesophageal junction, it is called Barrett's esophagus and is a premalignant condition to esophageal adenocarcinoma.

intestinal transplantation: Transplantation of the small bowel in patients with intestinal failure, defined as an inability to maintain nutritional status through oral intake. Transplants can be performed in adults and children. The most common indication in adults is short-bowel syndrome that is usually due to surgery for Crohn's disease, trauma, vascular accident, or volvulus. Transplantation should be considered in patients on total parenteral nutrition who have recurrent line infections, sepsis, repeated episodes of dehydration, cholestatic liver disease, or signs of portal hypertension. Immunosuppresive medications are required to prevent graft rejection after transplant.

intraductal papillary mucinous neoplasm (main duct, branch duct): A potentially malignant neoplasm of the pancreas composed of mucin-secreting columnar epithelial cells that create cysts, papillary proliferation, and varying degrees of cellular atypia. Main duct lesions typically arise in the head of the pancreas and have an approximate 70% chance of malignant transformation. Branch duct (*also called* side branch) lesions are typically seen in younger patients, found in the uncinate process or tail of the pancreas, and have a lower risk for malignant transformation. Most often, they are diagnosed incidentally during abdominal imaging. EUS with or without fine-needle aspiration is helpful in distinguishing low- versus high-risk lesions.

intrahepatic: A term referring to inside the liver. It often refers to the location of a bile duct branch or the location of a mass lesion.

intrapulmonary shunt: A physiologic condition in which the lungs are perfused with blood but are not ventilated appropriately, reducing blood oxygenation. It can be the result of pulmonary edema, pneumonia, atelectasis, hepatopulmonary syndrome, or pulmonary arteriovenous malformations. Shunts can be detected on echocardiogram with the introduction of agitated saline and the presence of bubbles in the left atrium in 3 to 5 cardiac cycles.

intrinsic factor: A glycoprotein produced by parietal cells in the stomach that is essential for the absorption of vitamin B_{12} in the small intestine.

iron: Atomic element 26; a trace element that is necessary for the production of heme and numerous proteins and as a protein cofactor. It is primarily introduced into the body through diet, and its primary site of absorption is the duodenum.

iron-deficiency anemia: Low hemoglobin as a result of inefficient bodily stores of iron needed for erythropoiesis. It can occur from dietary deficiency of iron or from acute or chronic blood loss, often via the GI tract. Endoscopy and colonoscopy are often used to locate a source of GI blood loss in this condition. Treatment includes oral iron supplementation, blood transfusion, iron infusions, and reversal of the underlying etiology.

iron overload: Pathologic state in which the body has excessive iron stores. It may be due to inherited disorders (such as hemochromatosis), ineffective erythropoiesis, accelerated hemolysis, repeated blood transfusions, or iron therapy. It can result in iron deposition in the liver (leading to fibrosis and cirrhosis, similar to hemochromatosis), in the heart (leading to heart failure), or arrhythmias. Treatment may include phlebotomy and chelation of iron.

irritable bowel syndrome: A functional bowel disorder that manifests as abdominal pain or discomfort and altered bowel habits without a detectable structural abnormality. The diagnosis is made based on the Rome II Criteria and usually involves exclusion of other causes first, including IBD and celiac disease. It can exist in diarrhea-predominant, constipation-predominant, and mixed forms.

ischemia: Inadequate blood flow to an area of the body either due to low circulating blood volume or decreased flow to the region, causing oxygen deprivation to the targeted tissues and organs and acute injury. It is often from disrupted blood flow as a result of vessel blockage or stricture but can also occur with severe dehydration or prolonged fasting.

ischemic colitis: Decreased blood flow to the colon resulting in inflammation and mucosal injury. Typically, it occurs in watershed areas (those areas of the colon located on the borders of arterial blood supply) and presents with pain out of proportion to abdominal examination, bloody stools, and fevers. Treatment is supportive, and most patients make a full recovery.

ischemic hepatopathy: Liver dysfunction resulting from a state of low perfusion and poor oxygenation, usually seen in the setting of sepsis or cardiogenic shock; *also known as* shock liver. It can be asymptomatic but may manifest as jaundice and significant elevation in serum transaminases, which may be greater than 1000 U/L (units/liter). Improving the predisposing condition usually reverses the damage quickly, without long-term sequelae. Rarely, it can lead to liver failure and death.

Ishak score: A modification of the Hepatic Activity Index used by pathologists to score the activity of chronic viral hepatitis in liver biopsy specimens. Activity scores are assigned based on 4 categories, with a maximum of 18 points: periportal interface hepatitis; confluent necrosis; lytic necrosis, apoptosis, and focal necrosis; and portal inflammation. Fibrosis is scored separately from 0 to 6.

Jagged-1: A gene located on chromosome 20 that, when mutated, causes Alagille syndrome.

jaundice: Yellowing of the skin or mucosal membranes as a result of accumulation of bilirubin in the blood, commonly seen in acute liver injury, liver failure, biliary obstruction, and hemolysis.

jejunal adenocarcinoma: A rare malignancy that often presents with abdominal pain, distention, nausea, vomiting, weight loss, or GI bleeding. It most often presents at an advanced stage because diagnosis can be technically challenging. Risk is increased in patients with genetic cancer syndromes, such as HNPCC and Peutz-Jeghers, IBD, and those with a heavy consumption of smoked or salt-cured foods.

jejunal diverticulosis: Outpouchings of jejunal mucosa through weak areas in the bowel wall. The jejunum is a rare location for diverticular disease and an uncommon source of GI bleeding. This condition can predispose individuals to small bowel bacterial overgrowth and vitamin B_{12} deficiency.

jejunostomy: A surgical procedure used to create an opening into the jejunum from the abdominal wall, usually for the purpose of inserting a feeding tube.

jejunum: Section of the small intestine between the duodenum and ileum. Its major role is in the absorption of carbohydrates and protein.

J-pouch: *Another term for* an ileoanal pouch.

juvenile polyp: A rare hamartomatous polyp of the GI tract, *also known as a* retention polyp, congenital polyp, or juvenile adenoma. Usually found in children, this type of polyp is 10 times more likely to be found in boys than girls.

Fenkel JM, ed.
Quick Reference Dictionary for GI and Hepatology (pp 109–110).
© 2014 Taylor & Francis Group.

juvenile polyposis syndrome: Syndrome that is defined by any one of the following: more than 5 juvenile polyps in the colon; juvenile polyps throughout the GI tract; or any number of juvenile polyps in a patient with first-degree relatives with juvenile polyposis syndrome. It may be inherited in an autosomal dominant fashion or can also occur sporadically. The polyps are usually hamartomatous and non-neoplastic; however, the syndrome increases the lifetime risk of colonic adenocarcinoma from 9% to 50%.

juxtaampullary duodenal diverticulum: Acquired diverticulum next to the ampulla that typically occurs on the medial wall of the duodenum. It is a false diverticulum because the outpouching does not contain the muscularis layer and can be a risk factor for biliary obstruction, bleeding, and ERCP complications.

kala-azar: A parasitic infection endemic to parts of India and northern Africa that is spread through the bite of female sandflies. It is also known as *visceral leishmaniasis*. Symptoms of infection include mucosal-based ulcers, hepatosplenomegaly, fevers, fatigue, anemia, and weight loss. Antiparasitic medication, including sodium stibogluconate, meglumine antimoniate, ureastibamine, and amphotericin B, may be used for treatment.

Kaplan-Meier curve: Statistical model used to estimate the fraction of patients living for a certain amount of time after a given treatment or intervention.

Kaposi's sarcoma (KS): A cancer of the lymphatic endothelial cells as a result of human herpes virus 8 (HHV-8) infection. It can be a rare cause of GI bleeding. It exists as 4 variants: classic, which is commonly seen in older Mediterranean or Jewish men; endemic, which is seen in younger men in Sub-Saharan Africa; HIV-related, which has become an AIDS-defining illness; and iatrogenic immunosuppression-related, which increases with the increased use of calcineurin inhibitors. Lesions typically appear on mucocutaneous areas as dark, purplish-colored papules.

Kasabach-Merritt syndrome: Profound thrombocytopenia, typically seen in children, as a result of platelet sequestration within vascular tumors, such as hemangioendothelioma or tufted angiomas. It is also known as *hemangioma thrombocytopenia syndrome*.

Kasai procedure: A hepatoportoenterostomy procedure typically performed as a treatment for biliary atresia. The porta hepatis is exposed and a limb of jejunum is attached to accomplish biliary drainage. Surgery is most successful when performed within

60 days of birth; however, in many patients, disease will still progress and liver transplantation will be required.

Kayser-Fleischer rings: Dark-colored rings encircling the iris of the eye as a result of copper deposition, classically described in Wilson's disease.

Killian's triangle: A triangular area of muscular weakness in the dorsal hypopharynx through which a Zenker's diverticulum can occur. The borders are composed of the oblique and transverse fibers of the inferior pharyngeal constrictor muscle and the cricopharyngeus; *also known as* Killian's dehiscence or Laimer's triangle.

Kings College criteria: Criteria described in 1989 to prognosticate which patients with liver failure required emergent liver transplantation. A different set of criteria was proposed for acetaminophen-related acute liver failure, which includes prothrombin time, arterial pH, encephalopathy, and serum creatinine. Nonacetaminophen-related acute liver failure criteria include prothrombin time, age, etiology, presence of jaundice, and bilirubin.

Klatskin-type tumor: Malignant biliary obstruction at the bifurcation of the right and left hepatic ducts, classically from cholangiocarcinoma. This type of tumor comprises 60% to 80% of all cholangiocarcinomas.

K-ras: A protein GTPase involved in the signaling of cell growth that, when mutated, increases the likelihood of cancer formation. It is most commonly associated with cancers of the pancreas, colon, and lung.

Krukenberg tumor: Metastatic tumor within the ovary. This type of tumor accounts for 1% to 2% of all ovarian tumors and is most commonly a metastatic gastric adenocarcinoma. Other potential sources include the colon, appendix, and breast.

Kupffer cell: Macrophages resident in the hepatic sinusoids that are part of the reticuloendothelial system. Functions include phagocytosis, development of liver toxicity, clearance of infection, liver regeneration, and immune tolerance.

Kupffer cell hyperplasia: An increase in the number of Kupffer cells within the hepatic sinusoids. This may be related to malignancy, such as lymphoma, systemic inflammatory disease, or thyrotoxicosis.

kwashiorkor: A malnutrition syndrome due to inadequate intake of protein with a reasonable total caloric intake that results in muscle atrophy and normal to increased body fat. The syndrome can manifest with a distended abdomen; dry, hyperkeratotic, or hyperpigmented skin; brittle hair; pedal edema; fatty liver; and hepatomegaly.

laparoscopic appendectomy: Minimally invasive surgical procedure to remove the appendix using several small incisions and a laparoscope.

laparoscopic cholecystectomy: Minimally invasive surgical procedure to remove the gallbladder using several small incisions and a laparoscope. It is currently the most common laparoscopic procedure performed worldwide.

laparoscopy: A surgical procedure that uses small incisions and a light with camera (laparoscope) to examine the contents of the abdomen or pelvis. Surgical instruments can be introduced into the abdomen through ports in the incisions and several minimally invasive surgical procedures can be accomplished using this technique.

laparotomy: A surgical procedure that uses a large incision through the abdominal wall to gain access to the contents of the abdomen and pelvis; also known as a *celiotomy*.

laryngopharyngeal reflux (LPR): The retrograde passage of gastric contents into the upper laryngopharynx and respiratory tract. Common symptoms include frequent throat clearing, globus sensation, cough, asthma, and hoarse voice. Proton pump inhibitors may help in symptom control.

lateral internal sphincterotomy: A surgical procedure by which the lower half of the internal anal sphincter is divided, creating a lower resting pressure of the anal sphincter. It is indicated for the treatment of chronic anal fissures refractory to medical therapy.

lateral pancreaticojejunostomy: A surgical procedure that connects a loop of the jejunum to the main pancreatic duct that is performed to improve drainage of the pancreas in chronic pancreatitis. It is also part of the Frey procedure.

Fenkel JM, ed.
Quick Reference Dictionary for GI and Hepatology (pp 114-120).
© 2014 Taylor & Francis Group.

laxative: Any compound that loosens the stool or promotes stool movement through the colon. This class of medication is used to treat constipation and may be given in oral or suppository form.

LC Beads: Gel microspheres manufactured by Biocompatibles UK LTD used in the transarterial embolization of hypervascular hepatic tumors and arteriovenous malformations. They can also be coated in chemotherapeutic agents and used to treat a variety of primary and metastatic liver carcinomas.

leiomyoma: A benign neoplasm derived from smooth muscle. Most commonly, it occurs in the GI or genitourinary tracts.

leiomyosarcoma: A rare malignant neoplasm of smooth muscle. Similar to leiomyomas, it is most commonly seen in the GI or genitourinary tracts. These tumors are characteristically resistant to treatment with chemotherapy and radiation therapy.

leishmaniasis: Infection with a member of the protozoal genus *Leishmania,* transmitted by insect vector—the sandfly. Four distinct syndromes of infection exist: cutaneous, diffuse cutaneous, mucocutaneous, and visceral leishmaniasis. Systemic, or visceral, leishmaniasis is serious and potentially fatal; *see also* kala-azar.

Leser-Trelat sign: The rapid and eruptive onset of multiple seborrheic keratoses (pigmented skin lesions) as part of a paraneoplastic syndrome. Most commonly, this sign is associated with GI adenocarcinomas but is also seen with genitourinary, breast, lung, and lymphoproliferative malignancies. It is named for German surgeon Edmund Leser and French surgeon Ulysse Trelat.

lichen planus: An immune-mediated mucocutaneous disease that affects the genitalia, oral mucosa, and flexor surfaces of the skin. The rash presents as flat-topped, dry, erythematous papules and can cause severe pain. The etiology of the disease is unknown, but it is associated with hepatitis C infection.

likelihood ratio: A statistical model used to assess the value of performing a diagnostic test based on the test's sensitivity and specificity. It calculates the ratio of the probability of a specific diagnostic test result in a population of patients with a certain disease to the probability of that same diagnostic test result in a population of patients who do not have the disease. A value greater than 1 implies that the test is associated with the disease, whereas a value lower than 1 implies that the test is associated with the absence of the disease.

linear furrows: Pitted, linear striations of the esophageal mucosa, a pathognomonic endoscopic finding of eosinophilic esophagitis.

lipase: A digestive enzyme that hydrolyzes lipids. The most important human lipase is synthesized and released by the pancreas. Elevations in measured serum lipase are associated with pancreatitis.

lipoma: A benign tumor derived from adipose tissue that may be present on the skin or within an organ.

liposarcoma: A rare, malignant neoplasm derived from adipose tissue. It most commonly arises in the retroperitoneum or thigh area.

lithotripsy: The destruction of kidney stones or gallstones with mechanical force, sound waves, or laser therapy. This technique can be performed externally or internally via endoscopic guidance.

liver: The largest internal solid organ composed of four unequally sized lobes and located in the right upper quadrant and epigastrium of the abdomen. It is vital to the body for functions such as blood filtration and detoxification, protein synthesis, lipogenesis, glycogen storage and metabolism, and bile acid synthesis. Blood is supplied dually from the portal vein and the hepatic artery and is drained via the hepatic vein into the inferior vena cava. Bile is drained through a system of ducts, called the biliary tree, into the duodenum to aid in digestion.

liver biopsy: Removal of a small piece of liver tissue for pathological evaluation. This procedure is commonly performed using a needle through the skin (percutaneously) with ultrasound guidance but can also be accomplished transvenously or during open abdominal surgery. Indications for liver biopsy include evaluation of abnormal liver tests, staging chronic viral hepatitis, and monitoring the response of liver disease to treatment. Common risks to the procedure include a greater than 1% risk of bleeding, infection, or injury to the surrounding tissue or organs.

liver cyst: A benign or premalignant encapsulated lesion of the liver that can be simple or complex. The majority of cysts are asymptomatic. Larger cysts can cause abdominal pain, hemorrhage, or compression of local structures and may require drainage or surgical resection. When multiple cysts are present, they may be associated with polycystic liver or polycystic kidney disease.

liver fluke: A parasite that, when ingested, can infect the intra- or extrahepatic biliary system, gallbladder, and liver parenchyma. The four major families of liver fluke that infect humans are *Clonorchis, Opisthorchis, Metorchis,* and *Fasciola.* Complications of infection include abdominal pain, cholangitis, biliary obstruction, and cholangiocarcinoma.

liver transplantation: The replacement of a native, diseased liver with a new liver. Liver transplant is a major surgical operation indicated for patients with end-stage liver disease refractory to medical therapy (decompensated cirrhosis), those with early-stage hepatocellular carcinoma, or those with fulminant hepatic failure, such as from acetaminophen-related overdose or drug-induced liver injury, who are unlikely to recover adequate liver function. It can be performed using a deceased donor (cadaveric) or live donor. Patients on the liver transplant waiting list receive organs in a need-based fashion using the MELD score to determine the patients most in need. The allocation of organs in the United States is governed by the United Network for Organ Sharing.

lobular inflammation: Focal inflammation in zones 2 and 3 of the liver or in the area outside the portal triad region that is predominantly seen in acute hepatitis and autoimmune hepatitis. Laboratory abnormalities, such as elevated aspartate aminotransferase and alanine aminotransferase, are often seen as a result. The presence of lobular inflammation as measured on the Ludwig-Batts scoring system suggests more active hepatic disease.

long-segment Barrett's esophagus: Esophageal columnar metaplasia (Barrett's esophagus) exceeding 3 cm in length in the esophagus that appears as a tongue-like discolored area of the esophagus on endoscopy, usually extending proximally from the gastroesophageal junction. Classification does not predict disease severity or guide clinical management. Biopsies are recommended to evaluate for dysplasia and cancer. Surveillance endoscopies are usually recommended in patients with this condition.

Los Angeles endoscopic classification: A scoring system for the endoscopic assessment of the severity of esophagitis, designated in 1994 at a consensus conference in Los Angeles. Grade A: 1 or more mucosal breaks 5 mm or smaller that do not extend between the tops of 2 mucosal folds; Grade B: 1 or more mucosal breaks larger than 5 mm long that do not extend between the tops of 2 mucosal folds; Grade C: 1 or more mucosal breaks that are continuous between the tops of 2 or more mucosal folds but involve less than 75% of the esophageal circumference; Grade D: 1 or more mucosal breaks that involve 75% or more of the esophageal circumference.

lower esophageal sphincter (LES): A smooth muscle bundle located at the gastroesophageal junction that is designed to prevent reflux of gastric contents into the esophagus via a contracted resting tone that relaxes during swallowing. Transient relaxations of the LES are thought to be the underlying pathophysiologic defect in GERD. If the LES does not relax during swallowing, it is considered hypertensive and a diagnosis of achalasia should be considered.

Ludwig-Batts scoring system: A histological grading system for liver biopsies used to uniformly assess the severity of chronic viral hepatitis based on the degree and patterns of hepatic inflammation (grade 0 to 4) and fibrosis (stage 0 to 4). The severity of inflammation is reflected in a higher grade. A higher fibrosis number suggests more advanced scarring. Stage 4 is considered cirrhosis.

lupoid hepatitis: *Another term for* autoimmune hepatitis. Its name is derived from the association of a positive ANA test, as seen in systemic lupus erythematosus, and autoimmune-mediated liver inflammation. However, patients with systemic lupus erythematosus are not necessarily at an increased risk for its development.

lymphadenopathy: The enlargement of a lymph node or nodes. This can be pathologic, as in lymphoma, or benign, as in a physiologic response to an infectious illness; *also called* adenopathy.

lymphangiectasia: Abnormal dilatation of lymphatic vessels, which can occur in the GI tract. Endoscopically, this can be seen as focal areas of white-tip villi in the small bowel without known clinical disease or as diffuse villous involvement causing chronic diarrhea and protein malabsorption (*see* intestinal lymphangiectasia). Focal areas are a frequent finding on wireless capsule endoscopy.

lymphocytic colitis: A subtype of microscopic colitis, a disease characterized by chronic watery diarrhea and normal appearance of the colonic mucosa on colonoscopy most commonly seen in middle-aged women. Biopsies are necessary for the diagnosis and typically demonstrate more than 20 intraepithelial lymphocytes per high-power field in the lamina propria, without thickening of the subepithelial collagen band. It is highly associated with concomitant autoimmune disease and celiac disease.

lymphocytic gastritis: A rare form of gastric mucosal inflammation characterized by the presence of intraepithelial lymphocytes. The mucosa may appear normal on endoscopy, so biopsies are necessary to make the diagnosis. It is most often associated with celiac disease and *H pylori* infection.

lymphoid hyperplasia: A pseudopolypoid condition that can be located in the GI tract, most often in the terminal ileum, whereby lymph tissue within germinal centers grows on the mucosa and gives a polyp-like appearance to the intestinal mucosa. This condition is rarely pathogenic itself, but it has been reported to cause intussusception. It can be associated with systemic diseases, including common variable immunodeficiency, colon adenocarcinoma, lymphoma, and infections; *also called* nodular lymphoid hyperplasia.

Lynch syndrome: An autosomal dominant inherited CRC syndrome characterized by mutations in DNA mismatch repair enzymes that cause microsatellite instability, a precursor defect in some cancer pathways. It is associated with an increased risk of GI, genitourinary, skin, and brain cancers. The Amsterdam criteria are used to identify high-risk candidates for molecular genetic testing. It is named for Henry T. Lynch, an American physician; *also called* HNPCC.

magnesium: Atomic element 12; an intracellular cation and enzymatic cofactor essential for energy metabolism, cellular replication, and neuromuscular activity. Deficiency can cause muscle weakness or cramps, fatigue, hypokalemia, nausea, vomiting, and heart failure. Excessive magnesium intake may cause diarrhea.

magnetic resonance cholangiopancreatography (MRCP): A diagnostic imaging modality that uses MRI to noninvasively evaluate the pancreatic and bile ducts. It is especially useful in the evaluation of suspected biliary or pancreatic duct obstruction and is highly sensitive to detect choledocholithiasis. MRCP does not require contrast enhancement and has largely replaced diagnostic ERCP in the evaluation of biliary obstruction, although ERCP may still be necessary to correct the diagnosed issue.

magnetic resonance imaging (MRI): A diagnostic imaging technique that uses a powerful magnetic field to align the atomic nuclei of cells to produce identifiable signals that are detected by a scanner and subsequently converted into 2- and 3-dimensional images. MRI is particularly useful in the evaluation of soft tissues, such as the brain, spinal cord, muscles, liver, intestine, and other solid organs. Unlike radiography or CT, MRI does not expose the patient to damaging ionizing radiation.

magnevist: A type of nonionic, linear, gadolinium-based intravenous MRI contrast agent used in examining blood vessels and body tissues with abnormal vascularity; *also known as* gadopentetic acid or gadopentetate dimeglumine. It is the most frequently used MRI contrast agent in history, with more than 100 million administrations worldwide at this point in time.

Fenkel JM, ed.
Quick Reference Dictionary for GI and Hepatology (pp 121-131).
© 2014 Taylor & Francis Group.

main pancreatic duct: The major excretory duct of the pancreas that drains pancreatic juices. It is joined by the common bile duct to drain into the second portion of the duodenum at the major duodenal papilla; *also called* the duct of Wirsung, named after the German anatomist Johann Georg Wirsung.

malabsorption: Inability to absorb one or more dietary nutrients across the GI tract, which can lead to malnutrition, anemia, and metabolic disturbances. It can be the result of an acute or chronic infection (such as giardiasis), an inflammatory condition (eg, celiac disease or IBD), small intestinal bacterial overgrowth, trauma, surgical resection, or enzyme deficiency (eg, pancreatic insufficiency or lactase deficiency).

malakoplakia: A lesion most commonly seen in the mucosa of the genitourinary tract but also found in the GI tract on endoscopic testing or other organs that is characterized by soft yellowish plaques or ulcers composed of histiocytes. These lesions are associated with an immunosuppressed state and are treated with antibiotics.

Mallory bodies: Large eosinophilic cytoplasmic inclusions in damaged hepatocytes, most commonly associated with alcoholic steatohepatitis and alcoholic cirrhosis but also seen in other forms of liver disease, including nonalcoholic steatohepatitis; *also referred to as* Mallory's hyaline.

Mallory-Weiss tear: A mucosal laceration in the lower one-third of the esophagus, usually at the gastroesophageal junction, as a result of severe retching or vomiting. The clinical presentation is of hematemesis after an episode of vomiting. Treatment is usually conservative, although endoscopic hemostasis may be necessary in severe cases.

mammalian target of rapamycin (mTOR) pathway: An important pathway in the management of immunosuppression, and a medical target for sirolimus and everolimus. The mTOR gene encodes a serine/threonine protein kinase involved in regulating cell growth, proliferation, and protein synthesis.

manganese: Atomic element 25; an essential metallic cofactor for the enzyme superoxide dismutase, a free radical scavenger in the body. A rare cause of abnormal liver enzyme tests, manganese toxicity (manganism) can cause irritability, apathy, gait disturbance, and Parkinson-like tremors.

manometry: A GI procedure that uses a pressure-sensing catheter to evaluate GI motility disorders. It is primarily used in the evaluation of swallowing disorders, incontinence, and suspected sphincter of Oddi dysfunction.

MARS: *See* molecular adsorbent recirculating system.

mastocytosis: A disorder of mast cell proliferation and accumulation that can have a cutaneous or systemic variant. In systemic disease, the increased release of mast cell mediators, including histamine, can cause abdominal pain, flushing, headache, diarrhea, arrhythmias, and bone marrow dysfunction.

maximum acid output: The total amount of gastric acid secretion 1 hour after stimulation with gastrin or a histamine analog. This measurement, obtained via nasogastric tube aspiration, is used in the evaluation of peptic ulcer disease, duodenal ulcers, GERD, Zollinger-Ellison syndrome, and other hypersecretory states.

McBurney's point: A location in the right lower quadrant of the abdomen, one-third the distance from the anterior superior iliac spine to the umbilicus. Tenderness over this area is classically associated with acute appendicitis. It is named for 19th century American surgeon Charles McBurney.

mechanical lithotripsy: A procedure accomplished with ERCP by which a gallstone that is too large to be removed from the bile duct with balloon pull-through and sphincterotomy is crushed using tools passed through the scope to aid in its passage.

Meckel's diverticulitis: Acute inflammation of a Meckel's diverticulum. Clinical symptoms at presentation are commonly indistinguishable from acute appendicitis and include abdominal pain, nausea and vomiting, and rectal bleeding. A nuclear medicine scan called a Meckel's scan can be used for diagnosis.

Meckel's diverticulum: A rare remnant of the embryonic yolk stalk consisting of an outpouching of gastric or pancreatic mucosa located in the distal ileum, usually occurring 2 feet from the ileocecal valve and affecting 2% of individuals. Most affected individuals are asymptomatic, although some may experience abdominal pain or rectal bleeding or have an intestinal obstruction. It is the most common congenital malformation of the GI tract and is named after German anatomist Johann Friedrich Meckel.

median arcuate ligament syndrome: The clinical presentation of abdominal pain caused by compression of the celiac artery by the median arcuate ligament (formed by the right and left diaphragmatic crura). It is frequently associated with recent weight loss because a fat pad that normally prevents celiac artery compression has shrunk. The diagnosis is made after excluding more serious causes of chronic abdominal pain and is confirmed by diagnostic imaging with duplex abdominal ultrasound; *also referred to as* celiac artery compression syndrome.

megacolon: A congenital or acquired condition characterized by extreme dilatation of the colon, often accompanied by colonic paralysis and severe constipation that may require surgical intervention. In the setting of ulcerative colitis or severe *C difficile* infection, "toxic megacolon" can occur; *see also* toxic megacolon.

megaesophagus: An abnormal dilatation of the distal esophagus commonly seen in patients with achalasia or Chagas disease in which partially digested and undigested food particles fill the lumen and predispose patients to aspiration pneumonia. Its formation is caused by absent or abnormal relaxation of the lower esophageal sphincter and abnormal esophageal peristalsis.

megarectum: A massively dilated rectum caused by neuromuscular dysfunction of the external anal sphincter and puborectalis muscle, often presenting as severe constipation and fecal impaction.

melanoma: A malignant neoplasm derived from melanocytes, most commonly found in the skin but also occur in the eye or GI tract. Melanoma is less common than other forms of skin cancers but carries a higher risk of metastasis and mortality. Melanomas can frequently be distinguished from benign lesions based on asymmetry, irregular border, variegation of color, and a diameter greater than 6 mm.

melanosis coli: A benign condition characterized by abnormal brown or black spotted pigmentation of the colonic mucosa noted during colonoscopy that is caused by the accumulation of lipofuscin-containing macrophages, usually as a result of chronic anthraquinone-based laxative use.

MELD-Na score: An alternate version of the original MELD score, the MELD-Na score was developed in 2008 to take into account the increased mortality of patients with chronic liver disease who have coexisting hyponatremia by giving added priority to patients with significant hyponatremia; *see* Model for End-Stage Liver Disease (MELD) score.

MELD score: *See* Model for End-Stage Liver Disease (MELD) score.

melena: Black "tarry" stools passed as a result of hemorrhage from the upper GI tract. The stool develops this characteristic appearance after being enzymatically oxidized in the ileum and colon. Hemorrhage from the lower GI tract (the colon) will usually present as bright red blood per rectum or hematochezia but not melena. The initial test of choice in the evaluation of melena is an upper endoscopy after achieving hemodynamic stability and volume resuscitation.

Ménétrier's disease: Enlargement of gastric mucosal folds caused by gastric mucosal cell hyperplasia. The condition leads to abdominal pain, protein loss, and anemia and carries an increased risk for gastric cancer. It was named after French physician Pierre Eugène Ménétrier; *also known as* hyperplastic hypersecretory gastropathy.

mesenteric ischemia: Inflammation and injury of the intestinal tissue as a result of inadequate blood supply through the superior or inferior mesenteric vessels. More common in the elderly, this condition can be caused by arterial embolism, venous thrombosis, arteriovenous atherosclerotic disease, vasocon-striction, or an episode of hypotension. The pathognomonic symptom is severe abdominal pain out of proportion with the physical examination.

mesenteroaxial: In the direction of the short access of the stomach, most commonly used in describing the direction of a gastric volvulus.

metabolic syndrome: The clinical association of several medical disorders that carry an increased risk of developing cardiovas-cular disease and diabetes. To make the diagnosis, an individual must have 3 of the following 5 risk factors: elevated blood pres-sure, abdominal obesity, high triglycerides, low high-density lipoprotein, and insulin resistance. Patients with metabolic syndrome are also at increased risk of having NAFLD.

metachronous: A term used to describe the identification of multi-ple primary (nonmetastatic) malignant neoplasms, particularly in the colon. A time interval must exist between detection of the first lesion and the subsequent detection of the second lesion (not synchronous).

metaplastic atrophic gastritis: Chronic inflammation of the gas-tric mucosa with associated glandular atrophy and subsequent replacement with intestinal type tissue. As a result, the stom-ach produces less acid and intrinsic factor, which can lead to vitamin B_{12} deficiency and anemia and can increase the risk of gastric cancer. It can be immune mediated (associated with per-nicious anemia), related to diet (particularly one with increased nitroso compounds), or associated with *H pylori* infection.

methemoglobinemia: A congenital or acquired condition char-acterized by a pathologic increase in the presence of methe-moglobin, an oxidized form of hemoglobin that cannot release oxygen to peripheral tissues in circulation. Patients present with shortness of breath, cyanosis, fatigue, and mental status change. Errors in the enzyme cytochrome b5 reductase are responsible for most of the inherited forms. Treatment is with methylene blue, hyperbaric oxygen, ascorbic acid, or an exchange transfu-sion, if severe. Acquired methemoglobinemia may be precipi-tated by topical benzocaine anesthesia that is not uncommonly used before an upper endoscopy.

microlithiasis: Biliary tract precipitation and crystallization to a size smaller than 5 mm, identifiable only on direct visualization with endoscopic retrograde cholangiopancreatography (ERCP) because they are too small to be imaged with conventional ultrasound or MRI. This condition is associated with acute pancreatitis, eventual gallstone formation, and sphincter of Oddi dysfunction.

micronutrients: Food-based nutrients that are essential for metabolism and are required only in small quantities, such as vitamins and trace minerals like chromium, copper, and selenium.

microsatellite instability: The occurrence of specific repeating nucleotide sequences in the genome (microsatellites) as a consequence of errors in the DNA repair process that predispose the underlying tissue to malignant transformation. It is most commonly associated in the GI milieu with HNPCC/Lynch syndrome.

microscopic colitis: A medical condition most commonly seen in middle-aged women that is characterized by chronic watery diarrhea and a normal appearance of the colonic mucosa on colonoscopy. It is diagnosed through colonoscopic biopsies and histopathology. Two forms exist: collagenous and lymphocytic colitis; both are associated with a high incidence of concomitant autoimmune disease. Treatment includes budesonide, bismuth subsalicylate, and aminosalicylic acid derivatives.

Milan criteria: A set of consensus guidelines by which patients with nonresectable hepatocellular carcinoma may qualify for liver transplantation. To meet the criteria, a patient must have either 1 hepatocellular carcinoma lesion smaller than 5 cm or up to 3 lesions smaller than 3 cm each, as well as no extrahepatic manifestations or obvious vascular invasion. Patients listed for a liver transplant also receive exception points on the MELD system if they fit within the Milan criteria; *see* Appendix 3.

Mirizzi's syndrome: Benign jaundice caused by obstruction of the common hepatic duct or common bile duct by large gallstones impacted in the cystic duct or neck of the gallbladder or by fibrous tissue obstruction in the setting of chronic cholecystitis. It occurs in less than 1 in 1000 patients with cholelithiasis and is treated by cholecystectomy.

Model for End-Stage Liver Disease (MELD) score: A scoring system originally designed to predict survival after transjugular intrahepatic portosystemic shunt placement and later used to determine urgency-based liver transplant allocation. It is a mathematical linear regression model that incorporates the serum creatinine, total bilirubin level, and INR for prothrombin time. The lowest score is 6, and the highest score is 40. The higher the score, the more likely a patient is to require and receive a liver transplant.

molecular adsorbent recirculating system (MARS): An extracorporeal liver assist device manufactured by Gambro indicated as a bridge to transplantation for patients with acute or chronic liver failure or as a bridge to transplantation or recovery in patients with acute liver failure. The system is connected to the patient's blood via a large central venous access line and has three circuits in which blood circulates: a blood circuit to remove water soluble and protein-bound toxins; an albumin/charcoal circuit to remove phenols, free fatty acids, bilirubin, and anions; and a dialysate circuit to regulate fluid and electrolyte balance.

morbid obesity: A condition of significantly excess body fat. The diagnosis is defined by a body mass index (BMI) greater than 40 kg/m^2. It is associated with an increased risk of developing cancer, cardiovascular disease, diabetes mellitus, GERD, gallstones, obstructive sleep apnea, osteoarthritis, coronary artery disease, and stroke. Weight loss surgery may be indicated if lifestyle modification and medical therapies are ineffective.

mucinous cystadenoma: A tumor with malignant potential that arises from the epithelial cells of the ovaries, salivary glands, and pancreas. Due to its malignant potential, surgical resection is usually recommended. Because the tumors are lined with epithelial cells, they often secrete copious amounts of mucin. Sampling of a pancreatic mucinous cystadenoma usually has an elevated CEA level.

mucinous cystic neoplasm: A pancreatic tumor with malignant potential, most frequently occurring in middle-aged women, that does not arise from the pancreatic ductal system. The tumors are commonly composed of multiple cysts filled with mucin, and surgical management is usually recommended.

mucosa: The innermost tissue lining of the respiratory, genitourinary, and GI tracts that is composed of epithelium and lamina propria, as well as a layer of smooth muscle called the muscularis mucosa when found in the lining of the GI tract. Glands within this tissue typically secrete the thick fluid called mucus.

mucosa-associated lymphoid tissue (MALT): Aggregates of lymphoid tissue involved in modulating mucosal immunity. These aggregates contain populations of B and T lymphocytes, plasma cells, and macrophages and can be found throughout the respiratory, genitourinary and GI mucosa. Rarely, malignant transformation of the stomach MALT can occur, often stimulated by *H pylori* infection, a process referred to as MALToma, or MALT lymphoma.

mucosal ring: An abnormal, thin, membranous, transverse ring of mucosal tissue usually found in the lower one-third of the esophagus that can lead to narrowing of the esophageal lumen, causing dysphagia or food bolus impaction. Endoscopic dilatation serves to disrupt the ring and treat the associated symptoms.

Muerhrcke's nails: Changes in the fingernails associated with hypoalbuminemia. White lines extend transversely across the nail bed parallel to the crescent (lunula). The lines do not move with nail growth and disappear when the underlying medical condition is resolved.

Muir-Torre syndrome: A variant of the inherited cancer syndrome HNPCC in which patients are at an increased risk of developing sebaceous tumors of the skin and cancers of the GI and genitourinary tracts.

Multihance: A type of nonionic, linear, gadolinium-based intravenous MRI contrast agent used to examine blood vessels and body tissues with abnormal vascularity; *also known as* gadobenoic acid or gadobenate dimeglumine.

multiple endocrine neoplasia (MEN) syndrome: A group of distinct, autosomal dominant inherited syndromes characterized by benign and malignant tumors of the endocrine glands. Type 1 causes tumors of the pituitary gland, parathyroid glands, and pancreas and may be associated with Zollinger-Ellison syndrome. Type 2A causes tumors of the parathyroid gland and pheochromocytoma and medullary thyroid carcinoma. Type 2B causes medullary thyroid carcinoma, pheochromocytoma, mucosal neuromas, and intestinal ganglioneuromatosis; patients with type 2B often have marfanoid phenotypic features.

muscularis mucosa: The thin layer of smooth muscle located between the lamina propria of the mucosa and the submucosa of the GI tract.

muscularis propria: The layer of muscular fibers located between the submucosa and serosa of the GI tract. It is composed of multiple distinct layers of smooth muscle, usually an inner circular layer and an outer longitudinal layer. This layer is integral in GI peristalsis and in the formation of muscular sphincters throughout the GI tract.

muscular ring: An abnormal transverse ring of mucosal, submucosal, and muscular tissue usually seen in the distal one-third of the esophagus. It can lead to narrowing and muscular spasm of the lower esophageal lumen, causing patients to experience dysphagia, and increased risk of food bolus impaction. Most patients with muscular rings are asymptomatic, but if symptoms occur or it is found incidentally, careful chewing and eating is the first-line therapy. Bougie dilatation can be used for patients with persistent symptoms.

***Mycobacterium avium* complex:** Two bacterial species that are difficult to differentiate—*Mycobacterium avium* and *Mycobacterium intracellulare*—and are important causes of opportunistic infection in patients who are immunocompromised, particularly those with AIDS and a CD4 lymphocyte count less than 50 cells/μL. Common sites of infection include the lungs and the GI tract. When in the GI tract, the most common symptoms are diarrhea, abdominal pain, and weight loss.

Mycobacterium tuberculosis: The acid-fast bacterial species that causes tuberculosis. It most commonly infects the lungs but can also affect the central nervous, lymphatic, genitourinary, musculoskeletal, and GI systems or cause disseminated disease (miliary tuberculosis). Within the GI tract, the terminal ileum is the most common site of primary infection, and the presentation can mimic Crohn's disease. Treatment is with antituberculous medications.

myenteric plexus: 1. A subdivision of the enteric nervous system; 2. A conglomeration of unmyelinated nerve fibers located between the outer longitudinal and inner circular smooth muscle layers of the muscularis propria throughout the GI tract. This plexus innervates the muscularis propria and helps control peristalsis. It is named for German anatomist Leopold Auerbach; *also known as* Auerbach's plexus.

MYH associated polyposis (MAP): An autosomal recessive inherited polyposis syndrome caused by mutations of the MYH gene (a DNA base excision repair enzyme). Patients commonly present in adulthood and are diagnosed by colonoscopy and genetic testing. The lifetime risk of developing colon cancer is almost 100%, and prophylactic colectomy is often recommended.

myotomy: The surgical division or incision of a muscle layer. In clinical practice, it is commonly performed to release pressure across a muscular sphincter, such as the lower esophageal sphincter for achalasia; *see also* Heller myotomy.

N-acetylcysteine: Antioxidant medication that is the antidote to acetaminophen toxicity and can be given orally or intravenously. It may also have some mortality benefit in acute liver failure from other etiologies.

NAFLD Activity Score (NAS): A scoring system used to evaluate the activity of NAFLD, taking into account 3 parameters on a scale of 0 to 8: amount of steatosis (0 to 3), amount of lobular inflammation (0 to 3), and amount of hepatocyte ballooning (0 to 2). Scores higher than 5 are consistent with nonalcoholic steatohepatitis (NASH); scores of 3 or 4 are indeterminate for NASH; and scores of 0 to 2 suggest against the diagnosis of NASH. Fibrosis is graded independently of activity.

naïve to treatment: A patient with a disease who has never received treatment for it; commonly used as nomenclature in patients with hepatitis C but can also be applied to other infections, including HIV or hepatitis B. Naïve patients have a lower incidence of viral resistance mutations.

nares: The two compartments of the nasal cavity, separated in the middle by the nasal septum. Colloquially, they are referred to as the nostrils.

narrow band imaging: An endoscopic technique that uses a limited band of light frequencies to enhance imaging of the mucosal surface of the GI tract. The light appears slightly blue and has been studied as an aid in the examination of mucosal lesions, including Barrett's esophagus and colon polyps.

nasogastric tube: *Another term for* NG tube.

Natural Orifice Transluminal Endoscopic Surgery (NOTES): An evolving method of performing abdominal surgical interventions by passing an endoscope through a natural orifice (eg, mouth, anus, urethra) and then using an internal incision, thereby eliminating the creation of an external scar and resulting in an improved cosmetic appearance postoperatively. Still considered experimental at this time, NOTES has been used in various applications, including transgastric and transvaginal approaches, to perform cholecystectomy and appendectomy.

necrotizing pancreatitis: Acute, severe inflammation of the pancreas that results in rapid cell death. This condition carries a high risk of pseudocyst formation, infection, organ failure, systemic inflammatory response syndrome, and mortality. Prophylactic antibiotics are often used for treatment, in addition to bowel rest, aggressive fluid resuscitation, and supportive care. Necrotic pancreatic tissue can become walled-off over time (*see* walled-off pancreatic necrosis) and require drainage.

negative predictive value: A statistical value used to predict the likelihood that a negative diagnostic test result accurately reflects the absence of disease. A higher negative predictive value correlates with a higher probability that a negative test result is correct. Negative predictive value = (number of true negatives)/(number of true negatives + number of false negatives).

nephrogenic systemic fibrosis: A rare, fibrosing disorder observed in patients with pre-existing renal failure who are exposed to gadolinium-based MRI contrast agents. Clinical characteristics include thickening of the skin with nodules and plaques and, in some cases, fibrosis of the internal organs. No effective treatment exists. Limiting exposure to and decreased dosage of gadolinium-based contrast agents in the past few years have significantly decreased the incidence of this disease in the United States.

neodymium-doped yttrium aluminum garnet (Nd:YAG) laser: A solid-state laser that emits infrared light. Historically, it has been used in endoscopy for inducing hemostasis of bleeding vessels, ablation of abnormal epithelium in Barrett's esophagus, and palliative GI tumor ablation but has fallen out of favor in light of more advanced endoscopic cauterization and ablation tools.

NG tube: A thin plastic catheter that is placed through the nose and directly into the stomach or beginning of the duodenum. Indications include gastric decompression in the setting of a bowel obstruction or ileus, medication administration for patients with swallowing difficulty, assessment of upper GI bleeding, enteral feeding, aspiration of gastric contents, and lavage of gastric contents; *also called* a nasogastric tube.

niacin: An essential vitamin, *also known as* nicotinic acid. Deficiency causes the clinical syndrome of pellagra. Supplementation is used for lowering body very-low-density lipoproteins and raising high-density lipoprotein. The most common side effect of supplementation is facial flushing, which can be decreased by taking aspirin prior to its administration. Dietary sources include beef, nuts, dates, avocado, eggs, mushrooms, and tomatoes; *also called* vitamin B_3.

Nissen fundoplication: An open, laparoscopic, or robotic-assisted surgical procedure used to treat or prevent severe GERD. Typically, the gastric fundus is mobilized and wrapped 360 degrees around the distal esophagus in an effort to strengthen resting pressure at the lower esophageal sphincter, thereby diminishing reflux into the esophagus. This procedure is approximately 90% effective in eliminating symptoms at 10 years postoperatively. Gas-bloat and dysphagia are the most common postoperative complications, and vomiting can be difficult to manage postoperatively.

NOD2: *See* nucleotide-binding oligomerization domain containing 2.

nodular lymphoid hyperplasia: *Another term for* lymphoid hyperplasia.

nodular regenerative hyperplasia: Benign, diffuse, nodular proliferation of hepatocytes, commonly associated with systemic autoimmune diseases, lymphoproliferative diseases, and myeloproliferative diseases that causes noncirrhotic portal hypertension. It can be diagnosed by liver biopsy showing an absence of fibrosis, despite imaging suggestive of cirrhosis; *also known as* pseudocirrhosis.

nonalcoholic fatty liver disease (NAFLD): The clinicopathologic condition histologically resembling alcoholic liver disease, occurring in the absence of alcohol use. NAFLD includes both benign hepatic steatosis and NASH. It is highly associated with the metabolic syndrome, but it can also be caused by medications, including prednisone, amiodarone, and tamoxifen. It is thought to be the leading cause of cryptogenic cirrhosis and may be diagnosed by ultrasound, CT scan, MRI, biopsy, or clinical suspicion in the setting of metabolic syndrome and elevated ALT. Treatment includes weight loss, lifestyle modification, and optimization of associated conditions.

nonalcoholic steatohepatitis (NASH): Inflammation of the liver associated with steatosis in the absence of alcohol use. NASH represents an advanced form of NAFLD, in which patients may progress to cirrhosis and end-stage liver disease, and is the leading cause of what was previously termed *cryptogenic cirrhosis*. It is graded using the NAFLD Activity Score. Diagnosis is made by liver biopsy in the clinical setting of elevated liver tests or imaging suggestive of fatty liver.

nonerosive reflux disease (NERD): Symptoms of GERD, including burning epigastric pain or chest discomfort in the absence of mucosal injury to the esophagus. The majority of patients with GERD have this condition. The majority of patients with nonerosive reflux disease are women, are younger, and lack a concomitant hiatal hernia. This categorization can include both acid reflux and nonacid reflux etiologies.

non-lifting sign: A term used to describe the feasibility of endoscopic mucosal resection of flat or sessile colorectal polyps during colonoscopy. Prior to resection, a polyp is injected with saline to lift it away from the surrounding mucosa. If the polyp does not lift, proceeding to endoscopic mucosal resection increases the risk of intestinal perforation. It may also be indicative of CRC invasion of the submucosa.

nonspecific esophageal motility disorder: Abnormal peristalsis or spasm of the esophagus that does not fit the classic manometric findings of achalasia, diffuse esophageal spasm, nutcracker esophagus, or hypertensive lower esophageal sphincter. It is often caused by GERD, and treatment is often initiated with acid-suppressive therapy. This condition requires esophageal manometry to make the diagnosis.

non-ulcer dyspepsia: Nonspecific GI symptoms, including epigastric abdominal pain, nausea, bloating, early satiety, and burning without any evidence of peptic ulcer disease or an identifiable luminal/organic etiology. It is also termed *functional dyspepsia.* It is sometimes caused by chronic *H pylori* infection that can be treated. An empiric trial of acid suppression is advocated for 1 month as first-line therapy. This condition can be exacerbated by anxiety, depression, and stress or be a side effect of medications, such as NSAIDs, antibiotics, or calcium-channel blockers.

nucleotide-binding oligomerization domain containing 2: A gene located on chromosome 16 that expresses a protein integral to modulation of the innate immune system through activation of macrophages in response to bacteria. Mutations of this gene have been shown to increase susceptibility to developing Crohn's disease; *also known as* NOD2.

null responder: Patients previously treated for hepatitis C who failed to achieve a 2-log reduction in viral load after 12 weeks of therapy. These patients are the least likely to respond to medical therapy if treated again.

number needed to harm: The number of patients who need to be exposed to a risk factor to cause harm in a single patient who would not have otherwise been harmed. For example, if a drug has a number needed to harm of 5, then only 5 patients need to be treated with the drug for one patient to have a bad outcome (ie, drug side effect). The number needed to harm is calculated by the formula: 1/[absolute risk increase (probability of risk factor − probability of control)].

number needed to treat: The number of patients who need to be treated with a medical therapy for one person to benefit from the treatment. For example, if a drug has a number needed to treat of 5, then 5 patients need to be treated with the drug to prevent a single patient from having disease. The lower the number needed to treat, the more effective the treatment is. The number needed to treat is calculated by the formula: 1/[absolute risk reduction (control event rate − experimental event rate)].

nutcracker esophagus: An esophageal motility disorder presenting as solid or liquid food dysphagia that can also be accompanied by chest pain. Most common in older adults, it is often treated with calcium-channel blockers, such as diltiazem or oral nitrates. Diagnosis is made using esophageal manometry with characteristic high amplitude peristaltic contractions greater than 180 mm Hg that often last for more than 6 seconds in duration.

obliterative hepatocavopathy: Occlusion of the proximal inferior vena cava that causes obstruction of hepatic venous flow and portal venous hypertension. It can be caused by thrombosis or membranous obstruction and is a variant of Budd-Chiari syndrome.

obstructive jaundice: Elevated serum bilirubin caused by intra- or extrahepatic obstruction of bile drainage into the duodenum. Most commonly, this is caused by obstructing stones in the common bile duct or compression of the biliary system by pancreatic head masses.

Octreoscan: *Another term for* somatostatin-receptor scintigraphy.

octreotide: A somatostatin analog used in gastroenterology to treat diarrhea, bowel obstruction, bleeding esophageal varices, and hepatorenal syndrome. It can be administered subcutaneously, intramuscularly, or intravenously. Depot doses delivered intramuscularly are also useful in the treatment of carcinoid syndrome.

odds ratio: A measure of association between an exposure and an outcome. It represents the odds that an outcome will occur given a particular exposure compared with the odds of the outcome occurring in the absence of that exposure. An odds ratio of 1 implies that the event is equally likely to occur in both study groups.

odynophagia: Painful swallowing, typically secondary to inflammation or infection in the esophagus. This symptom can be localized to the oropharynx, esophagus, or both and is not necessarily associated with dysphagia. An upper endoscopy is the first step in its evaluation.

Fenkel JM, ed.
Quick Reference Dictionary for GI and Hepatology (pp 138-140).
© 2014 Taylor & Francis Group.

Ogilvie's syndrome: Gross dilatation of the cecum and ascending colon in the absence of mechanical obstruction. Most commonly, this condition is seen in systemically ill or postoperative patients. It was named after British surgeon Sir William Heneage Ogilvie; *also known as* acute colonic pseudo-obstruction.

opisthorchis: A family of liver fluke parasites prevalent in Southeast Asia and Eastern Europe that can cause several GI issues, including cholangitis, biliary obstruction, and cholangiocarcinoma, if ingested and chronically untreated.

opsonin: A molecule that binds to antigens and enhances phagocytosis by leukocytes and macrophages. It is present in innate and adaptive immune response.

optical coherence tomography (OCT): A noninvasive, high-resolution imaging technique that uses light scatter to create cross-sectional images of the subsurfaces of human tissue. It is being investigated as a tool to better evaluate Barrett's esophagus and colonic polyps.

organoaxial: In the direction of the long axis of the stomach, most commonly used in describing the direction of a gastric volvulus.

oral rehydration solution (ORS): A solution developed by the World Health Organization for the treatment of dehydration associated with diarrhea. It consists of a solution of clean water, with specific concentrations of salts, carbohydrates, and electrolytes, and reduces the need for intravenous therapy.

Oriental cholangiohepatitis: A form of recurrent cholangitis characterized by biliary stricturing, pigment stone formation, bile stasis, and recurrent episodes of cholangitis. This condition is thought to be associated with episodic parasitic or bacterial infection of the biliary and portal systems. It is most prevalent in Japan, China, and Southeast Asia; *also known as* recurrent pyogenic cholangitis.

oropharyngeal dysphagia: Difficulty swallowing as a result of neuromuscular dysfunction or anatomical abnormality of the oral cavity or pharynx; *see* Appendix 13.

Osler-Weber-Rendu syndrome: An autosomal dominant disorder characterized by arteriovenous malformations (or telangiectasias) of the skin, mucous membranes, GI tract, and often the lungs, brain, and liver. It was named for Sir William Osler, Frederick Parkes Weber, and Henri Jules Louis Marie Rendu, who together first described the disease in the late 19th century; also known as *hereditary hemorrhagic telangiectasia*.

osteomalacia: A disease characterized by progressive softening and bending of the skeletal bones as a result of incomplete bone calcification and mineralization. Causes include vitamin D deficiency, malabsorption, parathyroid disease, and renal tubular dysfunction. It is also known as *rickets* when occurring in children.

osteopenia: Decreased calcification or density of skeletal bone with a bone mineral density T score between –1.0 and –2.5.

osteoporosis: Severely decreased calcification or density of skeletal bone, with a bone mineral density T score of –2.5 or less. This condition carries an increased risk of fractures.

oxalate: A salt of oxalic acid that can precipitate with calcium to form calcium oxalate stones, the most common form of kidney stones.

P53: A gene or protein responsible for tumor suppression. In its active form, P53 will promote apoptosis (cell death) of damaged cells. When mutated, there is inadequate apoptosis leading to unregulated growth of damaged cells or cancer. Inherited mutation of the P53 gene (a condition known as Li-Fraumeni syndrome) portends a significantly increased risk of cancer development.

pancreas: An abdominal gland located posterior to the stomach that has important digestive and endocrine properties. As a digestive organ, it secretes pancreatic juice containing digestive enzymes into the small intestine to aid in digestion. As an endocrine organ, it makes and secretes hormones that play a role in glucose metabolism and regulation of blood glucose. The pancreas is divided into sections called the head, body, uncinate process, and tail.

pancreas divisum: A failure in pancreatic fusion during early embryogenesis leading to two separate pancreatic ducts that drain separate portions of the pancreas. During normal development, the pancreas initially consists of a ventral and a dorsal portion that fuse to form one organ with one pancreatic duct. This condition is a risk factor for the development of pancreatitis.

pancreatectomy: The surgical removal of all or a portion of the pancreas. There are several types, including pancreaticoduodenectomy, distal pancreatectomy, segmental pancreatectomy, and total pancreatectomy. The potential indications include pancreatic tumors, pancreatic cysts, or complications of pancreatitis. Patients who have had a pancreatectomy are at an increased risk of developing diabetes mellitus or may

Fenkel JM, ed.
Quick Reference Dictionary for GI and Hepatology (pp 141-165).
© 2014 Taylor & Francis Group.

experience worsening of underlying diabetes mellitus due to the loss of endocrine pancreatic tissue during the excision; *see also* pancreaticoduodenectomy.

pancreatic abscess: An infected collection of pus that can form within or around the pancreas resulting from tissue necrosis and eventual tissue liquefaction. It is usually diagnosed as a complication of acute pancreatitis or abdominal trauma with cross-sectional abdominal imaging and is treated with aspiration, drainage, nutritional support, and appropriate antibiotic therapy.

pancreatic adenocarcinoma: The most common type of pancreatic cancer, originating from exocrine pancreatic cells. Painless jaundice is the most common presentation of tumors located in the head of the pancreas, which is also the most common location. Prognosis and treatment depend on tumor stage at the initial diagnosis. The most common surgical intervention in early-stage disease is a pancreaticoduodenectomy. EUS is often used to help determine the resectability of a lesion.

pancreatic ascites: An uncommon cause of ascites caused by a leak from the pancreatic duct. Analysis of aspirated abdominal fluid typically reveals increased levels of amylase and total protein. Treatment includes pancreatic duct stenting and symptomatic relief by paracentesis.

pancreatic cyst: A collection of fluid within the pancreatic parenchyma. Cysts are usually benign but some do have malignant potential. Most cysts are discovered incidentally, but patients may experience abdominal pain, early satiety, weight loss, nausea, or vomiting. Cross-sectional imaging is used to make the diagnosis, but EUS and fine-needle aspiration may be required to risk stratify a cystic lesion, particularly if it is more than 1 cm in size.

pancreatic duct: A hollow passage or drainage system allowing the pancreas to drain secretions into the duodenum via the ampulla of Vater; *also known as* major pancreatic duct, duct of Wirsung.

pancreatic duct leak: Disruption in the pancreatic duct leading to leakage of pancreatic secretions freely into the peritoneal cavity. This can present with abdominal pain and new onset abdominal distention (pancreatic ascites) after abdominal trauma, surgical intervention, or severe acute pancreatitis. Treatment includes endoscopic stenting, medical therapy, and drainage.

pancreatic duct stone: Calcifications that can form within the pancreatic duct, frequently in patients with chronic pancreatitis. Removal can be attempted endoscopically or stents can be placed around an obstructed stone to help relieve associated pain; *also called* pancreaticolithiasis.

pancreatic duct stricture: An abnormal narrowing of the pancreatic duct frequently presenting as postprandial abdominal pain, weight loss, and nausea. A stricture can be benign (eg, from chronic pancreatitis) or malignant and is usually treated with pancreatic duct stenting or surgical bypass.

pancreatic enzymes: Active components found in pancreatic secretions that help to break down fats, proteins, and carbohydrates. The term *pancreatic enzyme* includes lipase, protease, and amylase. Inflammation of the pancreas can lead to excess release of these enzymes, which can then be measured in the serum to diagnose acute and chronic pancreatitis. Deficiency or impairment of their release can cause patients to have steatorrhea, weight loss, and chronic abdominal pain.

pancreatic function testing: A diagnostic procedure used to determine whether pancreatic exocrine function is adequate by measuring response of the pancreas to create and release enzymes, such as amylase, lipase, and trypsin, in response to chemical stimulation by secretin; *see also* secretin stimulation test. Other types of tests, including fecal elastase measurement and provocative testing of para-aminobenzoic acid after bentiromide challenge, have also been used in the past but are not routinely available today.

pancreatic necrosis: A serious complication of acute pancreatitis in which parenchymal tissue within the pancreas may die or necrose and later become infected or walled off. Endoscopic necrosectomy is the treatment of choice for patients with infected pancreatic necrosis. Other management options include surgical debridement and serial percutaneous drains.

pancreaticocutaneous fistula: An abnormal connection that can form between a branch of the pancreatic ductal system and the skin. It usually forms as a result of abdominal trauma and frequently requires surgical repair.

pancreaticoduodenectomy: A surgical procedure, *also known as* a Whipple procedure, that is the procedure of choice for the removal of lesions located in the pancreatic head, second portion of duodenum, ampullary region, or common bile duct. The procedure consists of removal of the gastric antrum, first and second portions of the duodenum, head of the pancreas, common bile duct, and gallbladder. Since the invention of the procedure, a few procedure modifications have been made, with the most important being a pylorus-preserving pancreaticoduodenectomy that preserves normal gastric emptying.

pancreaticojejunostomy: A surgical procedure used to treat chronic pancreatitis that involves creating a longitudinal incision along the pancreatic duct and sewing the opened duct to a loop of small intestine (jejunum). This allows for pancreatic secretions to be emptied directly into the small intestine; *another term for* Puestow procedure.

pancreaticolithiasis: *Another term for* pancreatic duct stone.

pancreaticopleural fistula: An uncommon complication of acute pancreatitis in which an abnormal connection is formed between the pancreas and the lung pleura. The diagnosis is suspected in patients with unresolving pleural effusions and can be made by pleural fluid analysis revealing an elevated amylase level. Treatment is aimed at repairing the abnormal connection surgically or endoscopically.

pancreatic pseudocyst: A complication of acute pancreatitis thought to occur as a result of injury to the ductal system leading to a collection of fluid containing pancreatic enzymes, blood, or necrotic tissue; *see also* pseudocyst.

pancreatic rest: An ectopic focus of pancreatic tissue that may be found in the GI tract on endoscopy. The most frequent location is the stomach, where it appears like a submucosal mass that is slightly raised with central umbilication.

pancreatic sphincterotomy: An endoscopic technique that involves making a small incision in the pancreatic sphincter to decrease pressure in the pancreatic duct and improve drainage or allow better endoscopic access to it.

pancreatic stent: A straw-like device that is placed into the main pancreatic duct or minor pancreatic duct endoscopically to keep the duct open and promote flow of pancreatic secretions into the intestine. Stents can be of different size and are usually plastic. They are most often used to ensure patency of a pancreatic stricture from chronic pancreatitis or pancreatic cancer, but may also be placed prophylactically to decrease the risk of pancreatitis after an ERCP procedure.

pancreatitis: Inflammation of the pancreas that can be acute or chronic. Common etiologies include alcohol, gallstones, medications/toxins, or trauma; *see also* acute pancreatitis and chronic pancreatitis; *see* Appendix 23.

pancreatography: Radiographic visualization of pancreatic ducts after injection of contrast medium into the duct. It can be performed surgically, endoscopically, or radiographically. During an ERCP procedure, opacification of the pancreatic duct with contrast is called endoscopic retrograde pancreatography.

pancreatoscopy: A technique of direct visualization inside the pancreatic ducts using a fiberoptic camera on a specialized catheter inserted through an endoscope or via direct insertion of this small camera in the operating room. It is most commonly used in patients with intraductal papillary mucinous neoplasms being considered for surgical resection to ensure removal of all premalignant tissue but is also useful in resections of pancreatic adenocarcinoma.

paracentesis: Removal of ascites fluid from the abdominal cavity via a needle through the skin. It can be performed with or without radiographic guidance. Diagnostic paracentesis refers to the removal of a small amount of fluid for diagnostic evaluation, most often to assess for spontaneous bacterial peritonitis. Therapeutic or large volume paracentesis refers to the removal of a large volume (usually more than 1 L) of ascites fluid for comfort.

paraesophageal hiatal hernia: A more rare type of hiatal hernia in which the stomach and esophagus stay in their anatomic position but a section of stomach herniates alongside the normal anatomy in the hiatus, putting the patient at risk of strangulation. This type of hernia may require surgical correction.

parietal cell: One of the four major cell types located in the stomach's fundus. The parietal cell is responsible for gastric acid secretion via H+/K+ ATPase proton pumps in response to stimuli from G cells and enterochromaffin-like cells, as well as production of intrinsic factor needed for absorption of vitamin B_{12}.

partial nonresponder: A patient with an initial response to medication or vaccination with some clinical or biochemical improvement but does not reach the expected treatment outcome. In hepatitis C treatment, it refers to a patient who has a decrease of more than 2 log in viral load to interferon-based therapy but never achieves complete viral suppression on treatment.

partial thromboplastin time: One of the laboratory indicators used to monitor coagulation parameters. It measures defects in the common coagulation pathway and can be affected by blood-thinning medications, such as heparin.

Partington-Rochelle procedure: A modified version of a pancreaticojejunostomy (Puestow) procedure used to treat chronic pancreatitis. The surgical technique allows for the spleen and most of the pancreas to be spared. This procedure is more commonly performed today, replacing the original Puestow procedure.

Paterson-Brown-Kelly syndrome: The clinical triad of dysphagia (due to esophageal webs), esophagitis, and iron deficiency anemia. The cause of the syndrome is unknown, and it usually occurs in women. Treatment is aimed at correcting iron deficiency anemia; *also known as* Plummer-Vinson syndrome, sideropenic dysphagia.

peak acid output: A measure of the highest gastric acid production in the stomach in response to a gastric acid stimulation challenge, such as histamine or pentagastrin. It is calculated by adding up the acid output in the 2 highest 15-minute increments and multiplying the value by 2. Measurement requires a nasogastric tube and collection of all gastric output. Between 10 and 60 mmol of hydrogen ion per hour is a typical normal reference range.

pedunculated polyp: A raised colonic polyp that sits on a stalk. It is typically removed by snare polypectomy.

peliosis hepatis: An uncommon condition characterized by multiple blood-filled cavities throughout the liver sinusoids that has been associated with anabolic steroid use, azathioprine, HIV infection, and *B henselae* infection. It may present as abnormal liver enzyme tests, right upper quadrant pain, or hepatomegaly. The diagnosis is made by liver biopsy.

pellagra: A medical condition that occurs due to niacin (vitamin B_3) deficiency. The main symptoms can be remembered as the three Ds: dermatitis, diarrhea, and dementia. The treatment is vitamin (niacin) repletion.

pelvic floor dysfunction: A name for a group of disorders that occur when muscles of the pelvic floor weaken, leading to clinical consequences such as urinary incontinence, fecal incontinence, sexual dysfunction, or pelvic organ prolapse. Symptoms may initiate after childbirth or menopause or could be related to obesity. Treatment is aimed at strengthening pelvic floor muscles through retraining and biofeedback.

pelvic floor dyssynergia: Failure of the pelvic floor muscles to relax or paradoxical contraction of the pelvic floor muscles with defecation that can lead to constipation and anorectal discomfort. Treatments include biofeedback training, botox injections, and surgical management. Anorectal manometry is helpful in making the diagnosis and reveals the paradoxical contractions of the external anal sphincter during attempted relaxation.

pelvic floor retraining: An exercise program for the muscles of the pelvic floor that support the uterus, bladder, and other pelvic organs. Performing these exercises on a regular basis can lead to significant improvement in conditions, such as urinary incontinence; *also known as* Kegel exercises.

pepsin: A major protease enzyme involved in the digestion of food whose role is to aid in the breakdown of food proteins. It is released by chief cells in the stomach in its inactive form (pepsinogen) and is converted to the active form by gastric acid.

pepsinogen: A zymogen (proenzyme) of pepsin that is released by chief cells in the stomach. In the stomach, pepsinogen is exposed to hydrochloric acid, which converts it to pepsin.

peptic stricture: Narrowing of the esophagus that occurs as a complication of long-standing acid reflux disease. The strictures are usually benign but can cause dysphagia or food bolus impaction. Treatment is acid suppression and endoscopic dilatation if symptomatic.

peptic ulcer disease (PUD): Mucosal erosion and ulceration of the upper GI tract that may present with abdominal pain, GI bleeding, nausea, dyspepsia, or decreased appetite, usually caused by excessive acid exposure. *H pylori* infection and NSAIDs can also cause peptic ulcer disease. If bleeding, endoscopic treatment is often necessary. Otherwise, avoidance of NSAIDs, treatment of the *H pylori* infection, and acid suppression are the mainstays of therapy. The most common locations for peptic ulcer disease are the gastric antrum and proximal duodenum; *see* Appendix 15.

percutaneous cholangiogram: A radiographic test that demonstrates visualization of the bile ducts by injecting a contrast agent into the biliary system and imaging that contrast agent under fluoroscopy. It can be performed percutaneously or via an indwelling biliary catheter. The test can help identify biliary pathology, such as biliary stones or strictures. The percutaneous approach has largely been replaced by less invasive modalities, such as MRCP.

percutaneous endoscopic gastrostomy (PEG): Endoscopically guided placement of a feeding tube into the stomach that is indicated when oral intake is inadequate or in patients with an inability to swallow. An upper endoscopy is performed to ensure adequate GI anatomy and then a light is shined from inside the stomach through to the skin (transillumination) to select the proper place for tube insertion. Using a sterile technique, a plastic feeding tube is inserted over a wire through the skin and into proper position through the abdominal wall.

percutaneous endoscopic jejunostomy (PEJ): Endoscopically guided placement of a feeding tube into the small intestine that is indicated in patients with impaired gastric emptying and needed for enteral nutrition. It can be placed either directly into the small intestine via endoscopic transillumination or, more commonly, via an extension of a PEG tube.

percutaneous liver biopsy: A medical procedure in which a small sample of liver tissue is aspirated using a needle inserted through the skin. It is performed using a sterile technique and local anesthesia, usually as an outpatient procedure. Risks of the procedure include pain, bleeding, infection, and injury to the surrounding tissues or organs. Bedside ultrasound is helpful to minimize potential complications. Common indications for a biopsy include staging of viral hepatitis, evaluation of abnormal liver tests, or staging of fatty liver disease.

percutaneous transhepatic biliary drainage (PTBD): A medical procedure performed to allow drainage of bile in the presence of biliary obstruction or damage that prevents normal bile drainage. Using fluoroscopy, an interventional radiologist performs the procedure with a sterile technique and local anesthesia and gains access to the biliary system by inserting a needle through the skin and into the liver. A wire can then be guided to the desired location, and a drainage catheter is placed over the wire.

percutaneous transhepatic cholangiography: A radiographic technique performed to diagnose biliary disorders, such as strictures or leaks. A contract agent is introduced via a percutaneous approach, opacifying the biliary system and allowing visualization of the patient's biliary anatomy. Interventions can also be performed during the test if necessary (eg, stent placement or fluid aspiration for analysis). This technique has largely been replaced by less invasive modalities, such as MRCP.

perforation: An unintentional tear in the lining of the GI tract that is an uncommon complication of endoscopic procedures. It usually requires a surgical repair, although small perforations may be repaired sufficiently with endoscopic clip placement.

perianal: Nomenclature used to describe the region of the body located around the anus.

perianal abscess: An infected collection of pus that is located around the anus, usually as a result of IBD or a pilonidal cyst infection. Treatment includes incision and drainage, antibiotics, stool softeners, and underlying disease-specific management.

perianal Crohn's disease: One of several manifestations of Crohn's disease that comprises a group of disorders such as anal fissures, fistulas, abscesses, and anal canal stenosis. Perianal disease may be a marker of more aggressive disease. Multidisciplinary management between GI specialists and colorectal surgery is important in its management.

perianal fistula: An abnormal connection that forms between the anal canal and the skin around the anus that can lead to leakage of stool, abscess, skin breakdown, and ulcer formation. This condition is most often associated with Crohn's disease but may also occur after pelvic radiation or perineal surgery.

pericholangitis: Inflammation of the area surrounding the bile ducts. This finding usually refers to a histologic finding of inflammatory cells located around bile ductules, most often in the setting of systemic infection, such as sepsis.

pericholecystic fluid: Inflammatory fluid collection around the gallbladder that is one of the radiographic signs used to diagnose acute cholecystitis. In patients with chronic liver disease, differentiating between perihepatic ascites and pericholecystic fluid can be difficult, and the clinical scenario needs to be considered before making a diagnosis of acute cholecystitis.

Periodic Acid-Schiff (PAS): A histologic stain that involves staining tissues for glycogen and other polysaccharides. It is used to aid in the diagnosis of several medical conditions, particularly alpha-1 antitrypsin in hepatocytes and macrophages in Whipple's disease, and plays a role in the diagnosis of tuberculosis infections.

perineum: The anatomic region of the body that includes the genitals and anus.

peripheral parenteral nutrition (PPN): A type of nutritional support that is administered intravenously when oral (enteral) means of nutrition support is contraindicated and central venous access is not obtained. This type of nutrition comes in smaller concentrations so it can be delivered through peripheral access but is not an effective means of long-term nutritional support.

periportal: Nomenclature used to describe the region in the liver located around the portal triad. In the histologic evaluation of liver biopsies, periportal inflammation is commonly seen in chronic viral hepatitis.

periportal fibrosis: Deposition of connective tissue leading to the formation of a scar in and around the periportal area as a result of chronic periportal inflammation. With regard to staging of fibrosis, periportal fibrosis would represent stage 2 of a possible 4 in the Ludwig-Batts scoring system.

peristalsis: Intrinsic wave-like contractile movements of the GI tract using longitudinal and circular muscle fibers to propel food contents forward through the digestive system, starting in the esophagus.

peritoneal carcinomatosis: Metastatic spread of cancer to the lining of the abdominal cavity—the peritoneum. The most common types of cancers to cause carcinomatosis are ovarian, pancreatic, colon, and gastric cancer. Its presence typically portends a poor prognosis. Peritoneal fluid cytology, peritoneal biopsy, or surgical exploration and biopsy are potential methods to diagnose this condition.

peritoneal lavage: A diagnostic or therapeutic medical procedure in which a small incision is made under the navel to access the peritoneum. In diagnostic lavage, existing fluid is aspirated to assess for the presence of blood or fecal contamination, such as in a trauma case. Therapeutic lavage can be performed for saline irrigation or drug delivery, such as intraperitoneal chemotherapy in peritoneal carcinomatosis.

peritoneal signs: A group of physical examination findings that suggest irritation of the peritoneum from an infectious or noninfectious process. The commonly tested signs are abdominal rebound tenderness and guarding. Tenderness to percussion of the abdomen also increases the likelihood of peritoneal irritation.

peritoneum: A thin membrane lining the abdominal cavity and covering most of the abdominal organs. It is divided into 2 layers: parietal and visceral peritoneum. Irritation of the peritoneum by infection or inflammation can be painful.

peritonitis: Acute inflammation or irritation of the peritoneum that can be secondary to bowel perforation or abdominal trauma or be spontaneous in the setting of cirrhosis and portal hypertension. Patients typically present with acute abdominal pain, fevers, and nausea or vomiting and have peritoneal signs on examination. Treatment is aimed at the inciting cause, but empiric antibiotics and surgical consultation are standard; *see also* spontaneous bacterial peritonitis.

perleche: *Another term for* angular cheilitis.

pernicious anemia: The association of atrophic gastritis, parietal cell destruction, and lack of intrinsic factor leading to vitamin B_{12} deficiency and anemia. Intrinsic factor is a protein essential for the absorption of vitamin B_{12} in the ileum. Autoantibodies directed against parietal cells and the intrinsic factor itself are often present. Treatment includes vitamin B_{12} supplementation.

Peutz-Jehgers syndrome (PJS): An autosomal dominant rare disorder characterized by the development of intestinal hamartomatous polyps and a distinct pattern of mucocutaneous manifestations around the lips, face, and anus marked by melanin deposition. Although the polyps are benign, patients with this disorder have an approximate 15-fold increased risk for developing intestinal cancer compared with the general population and are at an increased risk of pancreaticobiliary and other malignancies. Most cases are due to a mutation in the STK11 tumor suppressor gene. Early diagnosis is important to initiate appropriate cancer screening for the patient and to screen close relatives.

pharyngoesophageal diverticulum: *See* Zenker's diverticulum.

pH monitoring: The traditional gold standard test used to diagnose acid reflux disease. A pH probe is placed transnasally into the distal esophagus to directly measure acid as a way to diagnose acid reflux or monitor disease response to medical or surgical treatment. pH monitoring can also be done without a physical transnasal probe using a wireless pH monitor (Bravo).

photodynamic therapy (PDT): A technique that has wide use in malignant or premalignant diseases, but within GI it is most noted for its role in the treatment of cholangiocarcinoma, dysplastic Barrett's esophagus, or esophageal carcinoma in situ.

The treatment requires 3 components: a photosensitizer, a light source, and oxygen in the tissue. Patients receive an injection of a photosensitizer. Then a specialized light source is used over the desired treatment area through an endoscope. When tissues are exposed to a specific light wavelength, reactive oxygen species will be produced that can cause destruction of malignant tissue. After the procedure, patients are photosensitive and require strict avoidance of ultraviolet light.

phrygian cap: A normal variant in gallbladder anatomy that can be seen in 1% to 6% of patients that is not thought to cause disease. It is often mistaken for gallstones on imaging and is caused by a fold in the gallbladder fundus at the junction to the body of the gallbladder.

phytobezoar: A bolus of indigestible plant material (such as cellulose) that becomes trapped in the GI system leading to early satiety, decreased appetite, and weight loss. It can be found in patients with impaired digestion or decreased gastric motility. Endoscopic removal can be attempted, but surgery may be necessary depending on the size of the collection.

pigment stone: A type of gallstone that consists of bilirubin and calcium salts. Compared with cholesterol stones, these contain less than 20% cholesterol content; *see* Appendix 26.

pill camera: A technique developed to enhance visualization of portions of the GI tract that cannot be easily accessed by standard endoscopic techniques, particularly the small intestine. It involves swallowing a small pill-sized capsule that contains a camera and wireless transmitting device. The capsule will then transmit pictures wirelessly to a data recorder that the patient wears during the procedure. The pictures can then be viewed on a computer. Pill cameras are commercially available worldwide.

pill-induced esophagitis: Inflammation, ulceration, or both of the esophageal mucosa resulting from the ingestion of certain medications and causing direct trauma due to their large size or by creating increased acidic exposure. Common medications associated with this condition are bisphosphonates, NSAIDs, doxycylcine, and iron tablets. Treatment is palliative with viscous lidocaine, sucralfate, and acid suppression, as well as cessation of the offending medication.

pillow sign: An endoscopic finding used to help differentiate lipomas from other GI submucosal lesions. The lesion is probed with a closed biopsy forceps, and lipomas characteristically have a soft, central indentation that is likened to a head resting on a pillow. This "pillow sign" is considered diagnostic of a lipoma, and a biopsy is not necessary.

placebo: A simulated or medically ineffective treatment that is administered to a participant in a clinical trial as a control in an effort to identify the true effect of the active medication given to a different participant. The benefit derived from the placebo treatment is called the placebo effect and is likely a measure of the patient's perception to being given a treatment that he or she believes will have benefit. The value of a new treatment is its effect above the placebo effect.

plasmacytoma: A plasma cell neoplasm that can occur outside the bone marrow and may be located in the GI tract. Patients can present with GI bleeding, bowel or biliary obstruction from the mass, or change in bowel habits. Solitary extramedullary plasmacytomas occur in less than 10% of all plasma cell cancers, but it should be on the differential diagnosis of masses found in the GI tract. Surgery may be indicated for obstructing or bleeding lesions. Multidisciplinary management with medical oncology is important.

Plummer-Vinson syndrome: The clinical triad of dysphagia (due to esophageal webs), esophagitis, and iron deficiency anemia. It usually occurs in women, and treatment is aimed at correcting iron deficiency anemia; *see also* Paterson-Brown-Kelly syndrome.

pneumatic dilation: An endoscopic technique used to expand a narrowed area in the GI tract, most commonly used for nonsurgical treatment of achalasia. The technique involves passing a deflated balloon over a guidewire with endoscopic guidance and inflating the balloon in the narrowed area for a specified period of time to weaken the muscle fibers in the stenotic area with radial force.

pneumatosis: A radiographic sign that refers to gas seen within the wall of the intestine. It can be a sign of ischemia, intestinal obstruction, or serious infection and requires a careful medical evaluation. Benign pneumatosis may also occur in patients who use positive-pressure ventilation for obstructive sleep apnea, had a recent endoscopic procedure, or have chronic lung disease, such as emphysema.

pneumatosis cystoides intestinalis: An uncommon condition in which submucosal or subserosal gas-filled cystic lesions are found in the wall of the small or large intestine. It can be a benign finding without an underlying cause, but may also suggest underlying GI disease (such as IBD or collagen vascular disease) or be a consequence of a traumatic endoscopy.

pneumobilia: The presence of air or gas within the biliary system. It is commonly seen after instrumentation of the biliary system during procedures such as ERCP. In the absence of prior intervention, spontaneous biliary-enteric fistulas must be considered, such as a cholecystoduodenal fistula in a patient with gallstone ileus.

pneumoperitoneum: The presence of air or gas within the abdominal cavity. Unless purposely created during a surgical procedure (such as a laparoscopy or PEG tube placement), it is a serious finding that suggests bowel perforation or infarction and should prompt surgical evaluation.

polyarteritis nodosa: An autoimmune inflammatory condition considered a form of vasculitis that affects small- to medium-sized blood vessels. It is more common in women and requires treatment with anti-inflammatory medications, such as corticosteroids. It occurs with increased frequency in patients with chronic hepatitis B infection and less commonly in those with hepatitis C infection. Symptoms include episodic abdominal pain, intestinal ischemia, fever, and fatigue. P-ANCA antibody is often present in the blood, and the erythrocyte sedimentation rate and c-reactive protein are increased.

polycystic liver disease: A condition in which multiple cysts are detected in the liver that can occur in isolation as autosomal dominant polycystic liver disease or as an extrarenal development of cysts in autosomal dominant polycystic kidney disease. More common in women, autosomal dominant polycystic liver disease can cause abdominal pain and distention and rarely is a cause of portal hypertension due to impingement of cysts on the portal or hepatic veins. Diagnosis is made using any abdominal imaging technique, and treatment options include draining cysts and then injecting sclerosing agents, surgical defenestration, hepatic resection, and liver transplantation in extreme cases.

polymerase inhibitor: A new class of direct-acting antiviral medications for hepatitis C infection that act by inhibiting the HCV NS5B polymerase enzyme, an integral part of the replication complex for the virus. An example of a medication in this class is sofosbuvir. Most polymerase inhibitors exhibit activity against all hepatitis C genotypes, although the response between genotypes can be heterogeneous.

polyp: An abnormal growth of tissue projecting from the mucosa of the bowel, most commonly occurring in the colon. Most are benign, but polyps may be premalignant and can be removed via endoscopic or surgical polypectomy.

polypectomy: Removal of a polyp. Most procedures are performed endoscopically, but they can also be performed surgically. Endoscopic polyp removal techniques include snare cautery, cold snare, hot biopsy, and cold biopsy polypectomy.

polyposis syndrome: A predisposition to develop large and numerous polyps in the GI tract. Most types of polyposis syndrome are genetically inherited (eg, FAP), but noninherited syndromes also exist, such as Cronkhite-Canada syndrome. A polyposis syndrome usually suggests a predisposition to cancer in the GI tract (or even outside the GI tract), so identification can improve survival through screening and early detection. Genetic counseling is appropriate for those with inherited polyposis syndromes who are considering having children.

porcelain gallbladder: A radiographic finding that refers to a pattern of gallbladder calcification that gives the gallbladder a porcelain-like appearance. It is thought to be due to a large gallstone burden and is most commonly seen in overweight women. It is associated with gallbladder cancer and, therefore, should prompt referral to a surgeon for cholecystectomy.

porphyria: An inherited or acquired disorder of the heme biosynthesis pathway (porphyrin pathway) in which certain enzymes can be affected, leading to acute or chronic disease. Acute porphyria is usually mediated via the neurologic system, and patients can have abdominal pain, nausea, vomiting, neurologic changes, and constipation. Attacks can last hours to days and are difficult to diagnose. Diagnosis requires specialized blood and urine testing. Chronic porphyria is usually cutaneous in presentation, with severe blistering disease, particularly of the hands, fingers, and face. Treatment varies by type of porphyria but may include phlebotomy, hemin, intravenous glucose and hydration, and avoidance of offending medications or stressors. Bone marrow or liver transplantation may be indicated in extreme cases of some porphyria types.

portal fibrosis: Deposition of connective tissue forming scar within the portal tract of the liver parenchyma only. With regard to staging of the fibrosis, portal fibrosis would represent stage 1 of a possible 4 in the Ludwig-Batts scoring system.

portal hypertension: Increased blood pressure through the portal venous system that is most often the result of cirrhosis but may also occur due to prehepatic disease (eg, portal vein thrombosis) or posthepatic disease (eg, Budd-Chiari syndrome). This condition is the underlying physiology for the complications of cirrhosis, including varices, hepatorenal syndrome, ascites, and fluid overload. If ascites is present, fluid and serum analysis revealing a serum ascites albumin gradient greater than 1.1 is consistent with portal hypertension.

portal hypertensive gastropathy: Changes in the gastric mucosa that are caused by portal hypertension. Endoscopically, the gastric mucosa develops a mosaic or snake skin-like appearance that can progress to mucosal friability, cherry red spots, and blackish-brown spots that are a potential source of chronic GI blood loss. Patients may present with anemia or occult blood positive stools. Treatment includes nonselective beta blockers and iron replacement. If severe, shunt procedures, such as a transjugular intrahepatic portosystemic shunt or a surgical splenorenal shunt, may improve the condition. Liver transplantation would also improve the condition but is primarily reserved for those with concurrent decompensated cirrhosis.

portal vein: A major conduit of blood to the liver, supplying more than two-thirds of the nutrient blood flow to the liver. It is formed by the confluence of the superior mesenteric vein and the splenic vein.

portopulmonary hypertension: The presence of pulmonary arterial hypertension in a patient with portal hypertension and no other explanation for the pulmonary arterial hypertension. It is a known complication of portal hypertension, affecting up to 10% of patients with decompensated cirrhosis, and can usually be reversed by liver transplantation if not so advanced that right ventricular dysfunction precludes surgery. It can be diagnosed by transthoracic echocardiogram if some tricuspid regurgitation is present or by right heart catheterization.

positive predictive value: A statistical value used to predict the likelihood that a positive diagnostic test result accurately reflects the presence of disease. A higher PPV correlates with a higher probability that the positive test result correctly identifies disease. PPV = number of true positives/(number of true positives + number of false positives).

positron emission tomography (PET): A nuclear medicine imaging technique that produces images of functional body processes. A biologically active tracer called fluorodeoxyglucose is injected into the patient, where it is taken up preferentially by tissues with high metabolic activity, such as cancer, allowing for better cancer detection. It is used to stage many malignancies and for cancer surveillance after treatment has been initiated.

post-ERCP pancreatitis: Acute inflammation of the pancreas that occurs as a complication of an ERCP procedure. The risk of this occurring is approximately 7%, and it is usually mild in severity. If sphincter of Oddi manometry is also performed during ERCP, then the risk of pancreatitis approaches 25%. Prophylactic pancreatic duct stenting may decrease the risk. It should be suspected in any patient with new or worsened abdominal pain after an ERCP procedure and is diagnosed by elevated serum lipase levels.

post-paracentesis circulatory dysfunction: A physiologic response that may occur after a large-volume paracentesis that presents as hypotension, tachycardia, acute renal failure, and sepsis-like syndrome. Appropriate plasma volume expansion with albumin can help prevent this complication. In patients with cirrhosis and ascites, removing a large volume of ascitic fluid can lead to asymptomatic hypovolemia. The physiologic response to hypovolemia is activation of the renin-angiotensin-aldosterone system with subsequent renal retention of sodium and water, which in turn can lead to complications such as impaired renal function and rapid recurrence of ascites.

postprandial: Occurring after eating a meal. Typically used to describe postprandial pain (ie, abdominal pain occurring after eating).

posttransplant bile leak: Leakage of bile occurring after a liver transplant, most commonly from the biliary anastomosis. In a live donor transplant or split liver transplant, it could also describe a leak from the cut surface of the liver. Percutaneous drainage of any collections can help decrease abdominal pain associated with this condition, but endoscopic or percutaneous stent placement is indicated. Placement of a t-tube can decrease the risk of bile leak immediately after transplant, but a leak may still occur when the t-tube is removed after 3 months.

posttransplant lymphoproliferative disorder (PTLD): An abnormal proliferation of B cells occurring after organ transplantation and often associated with Epstein-Barr virus infection. There are four subtypes of PTLD: early hyperplastic changes, polymorphic lesions, monomorphic lesions, and classic Hodgkin's type lymphoma. For early hyperplastic changes and polymorphic lesions, decreasing immunosuppression may be enough to treat the condition, but rituximab and more advanced chemotherapy are often required for the more aggressive types. This condition complicates approximately 1% of adult liver transplants but is more common in pediatric recipients.

postvagotomy diarrhea: Frequent loose stools that complicate approximately 20% of operations in which a truncal vagotomy is performed. Some patients may experience 20 loose, watery bowel movements daily that are unrelated to eating. The diarrhea may also be nocturnal. Dehydration and malnutrition may occur as a result. The mechanism is thought to be related to changes in gastric motility after vagotomy coupled with bile salt malabsorption and bacterial overgrowth. Treatment includes cholestyramine, loperamide, diphenoxylate, antibiotics to treat bacterial overgrowth, and possibly octreotide or surgery in severe cases.

pouchitis: Acute or chronic inflammation of the ileoanal pouch in patients after total proctocolectomy. Patients with this surgical history, usually with a history of severe ulcerative colitis or FAP, may present with lower GI bleeding, anorectal pain, or fecal urgency. Treatment of acute pouchitis includes antibiotics and anti-inflammatory medications. Chronic pouchitis may be improved with probiotics. If it occurs frequently, removal of the pouch and ileostomy placement may be necessary.

pre-eclampsia: A condition that can occur in the third trimester of pregnancy, characterized by hypertension and proteinuria. Liver tests may also be elevated. It is important to recognize this condition because if untreated it can lead to seizures (eclampsia), stroke, and placental abruption. The optimal treatment is delivering the baby, but if that is not safe for the baby, then bed rest, magnesium sulfate, and antihypertensives (with or without anticonvulsant drugs) may be necessary.

prepyloric antrum: The distal most portion of the gastric antrum, just proximal to the pyloric sphincter. It is a common site of peptic ulcer disease and *H pylori* infection.

prepyloric ulcer: Mucosal erosion and disruption located in the distal stomach, before the pyloric sphincter. The prepyloric region is the most common site of peptic ulcer disease occurrence. Biopsies of the ulcer are recommended to check for *H pylori* infection and to exclude gastric adenocarcinoma that has bulged through the mucosa, creating ulceration.

primary biliary cirrhosis (PBC): An autoimmune disease of the liver that leads to slowly progressive destruction of the small bile ducts within the liver. Over time, the liver becomes scarred, leading to cirrhosis and liver failure. The diagnosis is suspected in patients with a cholestatic liver enzyme elevation pattern, positive anti-mitochondrial antibody, elevated serum IgM, and liver biopsy findings of ductopenia or florid duct lesions. It is more common in women than men. Ursodiol can slow disease progression. Fat-soluble vitamin deficiencies, hyperlipidemia, and osteoporosis are also common in PBC and screening should be performed. Liver transplantation is recommended in patients with decompensated cirrhosis from PBC.

primary intestinal lymphangiectasia (PIL): A rare condition in which lymphatic vessels of the small intestine are enlarged, leading to a protein-losing enteropathy. It can be suspected in children with diarrhea, hypoalbuminemia, and edema and is usually diagnosed by age 3 years. Other complications of PIL include pleural effusions, chylous ascites, and pericarditis. The diagnosis is usually made by endoscopy and biopsy. Wireless capsule endoscopy is also helpful in establishing the burden of disease or to make the diagnosis if standard endoscopy is contraindicated or unavailable. Once diagnosed, symptoms can be managed with a lifelong low-fat, high-protein diet with medium-chain triglyceride supplementation. Patients with primary PIL have an increased lifetime risk of lymphoma, particularly in the GI tract; *also called* Waldmann's disease.

primary peristalsis: The first wave of esophageal contractions stimulated by food bolus ingestion, which helps food propel through the GI tract. This is in contrast to secondary peristalsis, which is triggered by stretch of the esophagus; *also called* swallow-induced peristalsis; *see also* secondary peristalsis.

primary sclerosing cholangitis (PSC): A chronic inflammatory disease of the bile ducts and liver with an unknown trigger that causes scarring and eventual bile ductular obliteration, which can progress to cirrhosis and liver failure. An autoimmune etiology is favored, although a specific target of immune activity is unknown. The diagnosis is usually made by imaging of the bile ducts showing pruning of the biliary tree with a beaded appearance on MRCP or ERCP. Liver biopsy can also be helpful in making the diagnosis and may show "onion-skinning" lesions representing concentric periductal fibrosis. Bacterial infections of the bile ducts are also common in this condition and antibiotic treatment with or without endoscopic management may be necessary. Patients with PSC are at an increased risk of having cholangiocarcinoma and IBD. Liver transplant is sometimes needed in patients with PSC and liver failure, although the disease can recur at a slow rate after transplantation.

proctocolitis: Inflammation of the rectum and distal colon either due to infectious etiology or a chronic inflammatory condition, such as ulcerative colitis. If inflammatory disease is limited to the rectum and distal colon, topical therapies such as steroids or 5-aminosalicylic acid enemas are often suitable treatment options. For infectious proctocolitis, stool samples and/or mucosal biopsies can help determine the etiology and treatment would be targeted to a specific organism. The diagnosis is made by sigmoidoscopy or colonoscopy with biopsies.

progressive familial intrahepatic cholestasis (PFIC): A group of autosomal recessive familial cholestatic disorders, of which there are 3 subtypes, that are caused by genetic defects in biliary transporters in PFIC 1 and PFIC 2 and by a hepatocellular phospholipid export defect in PFIC 3. It usually presents by age 3 months with pruritus, jaundice, and growth failure, but some forms may present later in adolescence. Ursodiol is used for treatment but usually does not prevent progressive disease. Surgical treatment with partial cutaneous biliary diversion or liver transplantation may be required. PFIC 1 is *also called* Byler's disease, named for Amish descendents of Jacob Byler, in whom the disease was first discovered. PFIC 1 and PFIC 2 have a low gamma-glutamyl transpeptidase level, whereas PFIC 3 has an elevated level. A genetic panel is necessary to confirm diagnosis.

prokinetic: A type of medication that enhances GI motility by increasing the frequency of contractions or by making them stronger. This class of medications is often used in the management of gastroparesis or chronic intestinal pseudo-obstruction; *also called* promotility agent.

promotility agent: *Another term for* prokinetic.

protease inhibitor: A class of medications used for HCV or HIV that directly inhibits viral-specific enzymes (proteases) involved in the replication complex of the virus. The US Food and Drug Administration approval of the first HCV protease inhibitors in 2011 increased the likelihood of sustained virologic response rate in genotype 1 HCV patients by more than 25%. HCV and HIV protease inhibitors are not interchangeable because they target different proteases in different viruses.

prothrombin time: One of the laboratory indicators used to monitor coagulation parameters. It is a measure of the extrinsic pathway of coagulation and can be used to monitor warfarin dosages and vitamin K status. Because factors involved in the extrinsic pathway are produced in the liver, patients with liver failure will often have a prolonged prothrombin time, and longer degrees of prolongation are associated with poorer outcomes.

proton pump inhibitor (PPI): A class of acid suppressive medications that block the proton pump located on the surface of gastric parietal cells, leading to decreased acid production in the stomach that, in turn, decreases the amount of esophageal acid exposure during gastroesophageal reflux. It is also an important class of medications in the management of GI bleeding and peptic ulcer disease.

pruritus: Medical term used to describe itching. Cholestatic liver diseases are often associated with the development of pruritus.

pseudoachalasia: A medical condition that mimics the signs, symptoms, and motility findings of primary achalasia. The most common causes are cancers located in the chest or at the gastroesophageal junction; *also referred to as* secondary achalasia.

pseudocirrhosis: Radiographic imaging of the liver that resembles cirrhosis with surface nodularity in the absence of histologic evidence of fibrosis or cirrhosis. Nodular regenerative hyperplasia is the most common disease that can mimic cirrhosis but diffuse hepatic metastases can as well.

pseudocyst: A fluid-filled collection similar to a cyst but lacking an epithelial or endothelial cell lining, usually occurring in the pancreas after an episode of acute pancreatitis. EUS with fine-needle aspiration characteristically demonstrates an elevated fluid amylase but a low CEA level in cyst fluid analysis.

pseudopolyp: A lesion or growth of regenerating mucosa surrounded by areas of mucosal loss with a filiform histologic appearance that is not malignant and is most commonly seen in the setting of IBD.

pseudopyloric metaplasia: A type of gastric epithelial change in which gastric glands are replaced by pyloric-type glands. It can also occur outside the stomach and is the most common type of metaplastic change found in the gallbladder and is seen in more than half of post-cholecystectomy specimens. *H pylori* infection may predispose patients to this condition.

pseudoxanthoma elasticum: An autosomal recessive genetic disease caused by a mutation in the ABCC6 gene that leads to fragmentation of elastic fibers in tissues. It usually affects the skin first with the formation of yellowish papular lesions, then the eyes, and later the blood vessels with premature atherosclerosis. It can involve the GI tract and is a rare cause of GI bleeding.

puborectalis muscle: An important muscle for anorectal continence, it is part of a sling of fibers that provide rectal support. Contraction occurs during peristalsis and relaxation allows defecation to occur.

Puestow procedure: *See* pancreaticojejunostomy.

pylephlebitis: Suppurative inflammation of the portal vein or any of its branches caused by intra-abdominal spread of infection, usually occurring in the setting of complicated diverticulitis or appendicitis.

pylorus: The muscular anatomic region at the bottom of the stomach that connects to the first portion of duodenum. It is a common site for peptic ulcer disease. Injections of botox into the pylorus may be helpful in controlling symptoms of gastroparesis.

pylorus-preserving pancreaticoduodenectomy: A modification of the original pancreaticoduodenectomy procedure, whereby the pylorus is preserved, allowing for normal gastric emptying. This is a common procedure used to remove tumors located in the head of the pancreas; *also known as* a modified Whipple.

pyoderma gangrenosum: Necrotic-appearing deep ulcerated skin changes that are thought to be immune mediated, often occurring in the setting of underlying IBD or serious hematologic disorders. The legs are the most common site for their formation.

pyogenic cholangitis: Recurrent bouts of biliary tract infection associated with intrahepatic pigment-type stones and subsequent intrahepatic biliary obstruction. Treatment usually includes antibiotics, endoscopic decompression, and surgical management, if needed.

pyrexia: *Another term for* fever.

quadrants of abdomen: Anatomical nomenclature in which the abdomen is divided into four quadrants: left upper quadrant, left lower quadrant, right upper quadrant, and right lower quadrant. This terminology is useful in describing where pain is located.

quadrate lobe: One of the four lobes of the liver. It is located on the inferior surface of the liver, more anterior than the caudate, under the right lobe.

Quincke's disease: A rare disorder of the immune system characterized by low levels or improper function of a protein called C1-esterase inhibitor. A genetic form is called hereditary angioedema. Presentation includes swelling of the face, airway, and abdominal symptoms. It is named for Dr. Heinrich Quincke, a 19th century German physician; also known as angioedema or angioneurotic edema.

Quinsy: A peritonsillar abscess, typically as a complication of tonsillitis. It is also spelled Quincy.

radiation colitis: Inflammation and injury of the large bowel (colon) caused by ionizing radiation. Patients at risk for this are classically those who have previously undergone radiation to the lower abdomen more than 6 months prior to presentation, most commonly to treat cervical or prostate cancer. Treatment may include antimotility agents, aminosalicylates, hyperbaric oxygen, parental nutrition, or diversion or resection, in extreme cases. Surgical management can be difficult after radiation injury and is more prone to anastomotic leak. The risk of a second malignancy in the colon is increased in patients with prior radiation exposure, and surveillance colonoscopy should be performed.

radiation enteritis: Similar to radiation colitis but with inflammation and injury of the small intestine rather than the colon. Treatments are similar to those for radiation colitis. Presentation includes diarrhea, weight loss, abdominal pain, nausea, lactose intolerance, and weight loss with an onset usually more than 6 months after radiation discontinuation. Intestinal strictures can also occur as a result and predispose to bowel obstruction and small intestinal bacterial overgrowth.

radiation proctitis: Inflammation and injury to the rectum as a result of prior ionizing radiation therapy. Commonly presents as rectal bleeding and can be acute (occurring within 6 weeks of radiation) or chronic (usually occurring more than 6 months after radiation exposure). Prostate and cervical cancer treatment is most implicated in its development. Diarrhea, difficult defecation, and anorectal discomfort can also be present. Endoscopic evaluation often reveals telangiectatic-appearing blood vessels in the rectum and treatment with argon plasma coagulation can often decrease the need for transfusions and improve bleeding. If obstructive symptoms are present, topical aminosalicylates and stool softeners may also be helpful in management.

radioembolization: *Another term for* Y90 (Yttrium) spheres.

radiofrequency ablation (RFA): A procedure in which electrical current is used to destroy tissue or cancerous cells. The energy is delivered via a small probe aimed at delivering the treatment directly into the target tissue. It is typically performed under the guidance of ultrasound or CT scan and is especially helpful in treating intra-abdominal malignancies, such as hepatocellular carcinoma. A small risk of tumor seeding of a RFA track exists, and careful attention to technique is necessary. RFA can also be used to treat luminal premalignant or malignant conditions, such as dysplastic Barrett's esophagus and carcinoma in situ of the esophagus. When used endoscopically, 360- and 90-degree attachments to the endoscope are available; *see* BARRX ablation.

Ranson's criteria: A clinical prognostic scoring system first introduced in 1974 to help predict severity of acute pancreatitis. It uses criteria from admission (GA LAW = **G**lucose >200, **A**ge >55, **L**DH (lactate dehydrogenase) >350, **A**ST (aspartate aminotransferase) >250, **W**BC (white blood cell count) >16,000) and at 48 hours after admission (calcium <8, hematocrit decrease >10%, negative base excess >4, blood urea nitrogen increased by 5, hypoxemia with partial pressure of oxygen <60, >6 liter fluid sequestration). Each parameter gets 1 point and scores higher than 3 are associated with severe acute pancreatitis and increased mortality; *see* Appendix 23.

rapid virologic response: A term used to describe a quick reduction in viral quantification to a value below the lower limit of detection within 4 weeks of antiviral therapy for hepatitis C. Achieving this type of response portends a favorable outcome with a high rate of sustained virologic response after treatment completion.

rectal examination: A part of the physical examination used to assess the anorectal area for irregularities, including masses, fissures, hemorrhoids, prostate abnormalities, and fecal impaction by stool. Stool can be obtained during a rectal examination to test for occult blood or infection. It is regularly performed with the physician wearing gloves and using lubricating jelly. Digital rectal examination is not recommended alone or in combination with fecal occult blood testing as a sufficient screening tool for colon cancer; *also called* a digital rectal examination.

rectal prolapse: A medical condition in which the rectum protrudes through the anus and becomes externalized, particularly in the setting of Valsalva maneuvers such as defecation. It is more common in women but can occur in men and is thought to occur from the weakening of pelvic floor muscles. It may present with rectal bleeding and is often confused for hemorrhoids. Treatment includes prevention of constipation and surgical correction of more advanced or symptomatic cases.

rectoanal inhibitory reflex: The natural decrease in pressure of the internal anal sphincter in response to increased rectal pressure. It can be tested by inflating a balloon in the rectum and measuring basal pressure across the sphincter. Normal physiology is a decrease of 25% or more in basal pressure across the sphincter, with rapid return to normal pressure after deflation. This reflex is absent in Hirschsprung's disease.

rectocele: A common defect of the pelvic floor caused by thinning of the rectovaginal septum in which the anterior wall of the rectum bulges into the posterior wall of the vagina. Childbirth, chronic constipation, and colorectal surgery can be predisposing factors. Diagnosis is made using defecography, and treatment can be medical or surgical depending on the severity.

rectovaginal fistula: An abnormal communication or connection between the rectum and the vagina allowing for the passage of material between the two organs. Within gastroenterology, it most often occurs in fistulizing Crohn's disease but can also result from childbirth trauma or radiation treatment or as a complication of a pelvic malignancy. Treatment may include surgery or medical therapy, depending on the predisposing condition.

rectovesical fistula: An abnormal communication or connection between the rectum and the bladder allowing for the passage of material between the two organs. Symptoms can include pneumaturia, which is the presence of bubbles or passage of air in the urine, or frequent urinary tract infections. It can occur as a complication of IBD, complicated diverticulitis, colorectal carcinoma, or pelvic radiation therapy. Treatment may include surgery or medical therapy aimed at correcting the underlying condition.

recurrent pyogenic cholangitis: *See* Oriental cholangiohepatitis.

refeeding syndrome: A metabolic disorder in which life-threatening fluid and electrolyte shifts may occur when initiating nutritional support to a patient who is severely malnourished. Common findings include low serum levels of phosphorus, potassium, and magnesium, but trace minerals and vitamins including thiamine can also be diminished. The pathophysiology of refeeding syndrome involves insulin secretion in response to carbohydrate introduction that drives the above electrolytes intracellularly leading to low serum concentrations. Patients who are malnourished already have a reduced electrolyte reserve and are most susceptible to this phenomenon. Consequences of refeeding syndrome may include cardiac arrest, respiratory failure, congestive heart failure, altered mental status, seizures, and weakness. To prevent this syndrome, identification of those at risk before initiating feeding, slow introduction of feeding, close electrolyte monitoring, and vitamin support with thiamine is key. *See also* anorexia nervosa.

reflux esophagitis: Inflammation of the esophageal mucosa as a result of GERD. It often presents as heartburn, chest pain, or odynophagia. Untreated, it can predispose individuals to Barrett's esophagus, esophageal cancer, and esophageal strictures. Lifestyle modification and acid suppression with H2 blockers or proton pump inhibitors are the mainstays of treatment.

refractory sprue: Celiac disease that does not improve after at least 6 to 12 months of a gluten-free diet. It can be further divided into Type 1 and 2. In Type 1, the intraepithelial lymphocyte population is polyclonal, and this type often responds to immunosuppressive mediations like corticosteroids. Type 2 has a monoclonal population of lymphocytes and portends a higher risk to the development of intestinal T-cell lymphoma.

regional enteritis: *Another term for* Crohn's disease.

relapse (r): A term used to describe the recurrence of a disease after it was thought to have been cured. In gastroenterology, this term is often used to describe the recurrence of hepatitis C infection within 6 months of completing antiviral treatment when the patient had complete viral suppression during treatment. Knowledge of prior treatment attempts is important in determining the retreatment strategy with regard to medication choice and treatment duration.

relative risk reduction: An epidemiologic calculation determined by dividing the absolute risk reduction by the control event rate. For example, if a disease is present in 20% of participants but only present in 5% of participants receiving an experimental medication, then the relative risk reduction would be the following (20% − 5%)/20% = 75%.

replaced right hepatic artery: An anatomical variant where the right hepatic artery arises from a location other than its normal origin in the celiac trunk, typically the superior mesenteric artery. It is the most common hepatic arterial variation and is present in approximately 10% of all people. Knowing the location of the right hepatic artery is important in planning for abdominal surgeries involving the liver, particularly liver transplantation.

response-guided therapy: The concept that the duration of medical therapy can be tailored to an individual patient's response to the therapy. This concept is the cornerstone of antiviral therapy for individuals with hepatitis C who are naïve to treatment or were previous relapsers or partial responders. Patients who achieve extended rapid virologic response are eligible for shortened therapy, whereas patients who are slower to respond are treated for a longer duration.

reticulin stain: A histological stain used on pathologic specimens that stains tissue containing type III collagen fibers (reticulin). These fibers form much of the basic pericellular structure in the liver, and patterns of injury to the liver can often be determined based on the distribution or pattern of reticulin fiber staining seen on histology, making it a useful stain in hepatology.

Reynolds' pentad: The five symptoms and signs of ascending cholangitis are abdominal pain, fever, and jaundice (known as Charcot's triad); shock (low blood pressure); and change in mental status. This association may increase detection of ascending cholangitis and improve outcome via early detection.

riboflavin: Another name for vitamin B_2, an important micronutrient found in eggs, milk, cheese, and wheat bran that is used by many cellular targets, including flavoproteins (flavin adenine dinucleotide and flavin mononucleotide). It is responsible for the yellow/red color of B vitamin solutions. Deficiency, which can occur in IBD, HIV, and women taking oral contraceptive agents, can cause anemia, photophobia, dermatitis (particularly of the scrotum), and angular cheilitis.

Rockall score: A scoring system used to predict prognosis and risk of mortality in patients with acute upper GI bleeding and can be clinically useful in helping to determine which patients require inpatient versus outpatient monitoring. The score ranges from 0 to 11 and a score less than 3 predicts a favorable prognosis. Five components comprise the score, which can be remembered by the mnemonic ABCDE (*A*ge, *B*lood pressure drop [shock], *C*omorbidities, *D*iagnosis of bleeding, and *E*ndoscopic stigmata).

Rome criteria: Expert consensus criteria developed to better define and diagnose functional GI disorders (those disorders that cannot be explained based on the presence of structural or tissue abnormalities). The criteria rely on clinical symptoms to classify functional GI disorders, such as IBD, functional heartburn, and functional abdominal pain. The criteria underwent a third revision in 2006. Web site: www.romecriteria.org

Roth net: An endoscopic tool used to retrieve foreign objects, such as an impacted food bolus or large polyps, after they have been excised. It is placed into the working channel of a flexible endoscope and can be opened and closed by an operator outside the patient. The entire scope needs to be withdrawn to remove the object captured inside the net with the net in the closed position.

Rotor syndrome: An autosomal recessive genetic disorder of hepatic bilirubin clearance leading to increased levels of conjugated bilirubin in the blood stream and the clinical presentation of jaundice and occasional pruritus. The specific enzyme defect is not currently known, but it is thought to be a benign condition and requires no specific treatment. It is not associated with the development of fibrosis or cirrhosis. It can be distinguished from Dubin-Johnson syndrome by measuring urinary total coproporphyrin concentrations, which are usually elevated in Rotor syndome but are not in Dubin-Johnson syndrome.

Roux-en-Y gastric bypass: A common form of bariatric (weight loss) surgery that involves a Y-shaped anastomosis of jejunum to a portion of the stomach, which has been divided into a small pouch and an excluded portion. This operation promotes weight loss via several mechanisms, including restriction of food intake via the small gastric pouch and fat malabsorption. Most patients lose 50% to 80% of their excess body weight, although results can vary depending on dietary compliance after the procedure. Patients typically require multivitamin and iron supplementation. Posthumously named after Swiss surgeon Cesar Roux.

Roux-en-Y hepaticojejunostomy: A surgical procedure used to treat benign and malignant biliary tract abnormalities, including obstructing pancreatic cancer, biliary strictures, or choledochal cysts. During the operation, a loop of jejunum (Roux limb) is mobilized and anastomosed to the common hepatic duct to obtain biliary drainage. This technique is also used in many liver transplant operations, particularly in live donor transplant where only one of the donor hepatic ducts is available for anastomosis or in patients with primary sclerosing cholangitis who have disease of the native common bile duct.

Roux limb: A segment of jejunum created in a Roux-en-Y gastric bypass or hepaticojejunostomy. The length of the limb has a direct impact on the amount of weight loss and the amount of malabsorption during a bypass procedure and can vary between 80 and 150 cm.

rubber band ligation: An endoscopic or proctoscopic technique where a taut rubber band is placed around an undesired vascular structure, such as a hemorrhoid or varix, cutting off its blood supply to allow for decompression or obliteration and ultimately decreasing the risk of hemorrhage and discomfort.

Ruvalcaba-Myhre-Smith syndrome: A rare autosomal dominant condition with diffuse hamartomatous GI polyp formation associated with delayed development, muscle disorders, lipomas (growths consisting of fat tissue), and neurological sequelae, such as macrocephaly. Recently, it was recategorized as a PHTS called Banayan Ruvalcaba Riley syndrome.

S

sacral nerve stimulation: Manipulation of the sacral nerve using an electrical current supplied by an implanted device to improve symptoms associated with fecal or urinary incontinence, interstitial cystitis, and chronic pelvic pain. The device is usually implanted into the lower abdomen and is referred to as sacral neuromodulation.

sacroiliitis: Inflammation of the joint connecting the sacrum (lower spine) to the ilium (pelvis) in the lower back causing back pain that can radiate into the legs. This condition is associated with IBD and other HLA B27–associated spondyloarthropathies, including ankylosing spondylitis.

saliva: A watery solution produced in the salivary glands that is composed mostly of water, electrolytes, mucus, and digestive enzymes and plays important roles in food lubrication and initial enzymatic digestion. Salivary glands make more than 2 pints of saliva per day. Saliva also helps prevent tooth decay.

salivary pooling: The accumulation of saliva in the mouth and oropharynx, which can be normal to some extent. Excessive pooling may be a sign of an oropharyngeal carcinoma or a motor/swallowing disorder, such as amyotrophic lateral sclerosis.

Salmonella: A gram-negative bacteria responsible for several illness in humans, including typhoid fever and invasive foodborne gastroenteritis. Blood stream infection with *Salmonella* can also occur in patients who are immunocompromised, including those with sickle cell disease. Treatment is usually supportive, but antibiotic treatment with a fluoroquinolone or third-generation cephalosporin is indicated in those with severe infection or those at risk of severe infection, such as infants and elderly individuals.

Fenkel JM, ed.
Quick Reference Dictionary for GI and Hepatology (pp 175-191).
© 2014 Taylor & Francis Group.

sarcoidosis: A chronic inflammatory disorder characterized by the formation of non-necrotizing granulomas, most commonly in the lung and mediastinal lymph nodes. It can also affect the GI tract, presenting as abdominal pain, bloating, or weight loss and can involve the liver, causing cirrhosis and liver failure. Treatment is primarily with corticosteroids, although research efforts are being directed at its pathophysiology and treatment because its mechanism is poorly understood.

Savary dilator: A type of endoscopic device used to dilate a stricture in the upper GI tract in which a dilator is passed over a guidewire that has been positioned with or without fluoroscopic guidance. It has also been called the *Savary-Gilliard dilator*.

Savary-Miller classification: A scoring system aimed to standardize reporting of erosive esophagitis caused by GERD. There are five classes of esophagitis in this system: V is the appearance of Barrett's esophagus, whereas classes I to IV describe increasing degrees of esophageal inflammation and erosion.

Schatzki ring: A benign, mucosal, diaphragm-like ring of tissue usually located in the distal esophagus near the gastroesophageal junction that may be a cause of dysphagia or food bolus impaction requiring endoscopic dilatation. It may also be detected incidentally on an upper endoscopy and be asymptomatic. The rings may recur after dilatation and retreatment may be necessary. If recurrence is quick or frequent, investigation for esophageal motility disorders should be considered.

Schilling test: A diagnostic test used to investigate for pernicious anemia as a cause of vitamin B_{12} deficiency. After an overnight fast, a patient receives an intramuscular injection of vitamin B_{12} to ensure saturation of the body's B_{12} stores. Next, radiolabeled vitamin B_{12} is given orally. Because the body has saturated stores of B_{12}, this labeled B_{12} should all be excreted in the urine if it is absorbed properly, so urinary concentrations are measured at 24 hours and less than 10% excretion is suspicious for pernicious anemia. The test is then repeated, giving the patient radiolabeled B_{12} and oral intrinsic factor, which should increase urinary excretion. The test may also be performed giving consecutive doses of B_{12} labeled with different isotopes, one with intrinsic factor and one without, and then the ratio of the isotopes can be compared with diagnosed pernicious anemia.

Schistosomiasis: A parasitic disease caused by a trematode worm that can live in selected freshwater snails in Africa, the Middle East, Southeast Asia, South America, and rarely the Caribbean. It is also known as *bilharzia*. Humans become infected when their skin contacts contaminated water. Disease symptoms are mainly due to the body's response to the worms leading to inflammation in the skin, GI tract, liver, spleen, lungs, and bladder. Testing the blood, stool, or urine for its presence can make the diagnosis. Treatment is praziquantel, but damage caused by the inflammatory response may not be fixed by eradicating the parasite.

schwannoma: A benign tumor of the outer layer of nerves composed of Schwann cells that normally help form the outer myelin sheath of nerves. These rare tumors can occur in the GI tract and are on the differential diagnosis for subepithelial masses found incidentally on endoscopy.

sclerotherapy: An endoscopic technique used to treat bleeding esophageal varices or prevent hemorrhage from varices with high risk stigmata whereby a sclerosing agent, such as ethanolamine, is injected into a varix through an endoscope under direct visualization. This technique has largely been replaced by endoscopic band ligation in the United States, but remains an effective tool in cases where band ligation is unsuccessful or unavailable. Patients may experience chest pain, fevers, odynophagia, or develop mediastinitis or esophageal strictures as a result of the procedure.

Seattle protocol: A systematic approach to surveillance of Barrett's esophagus by taking biopsies in four quadrants every 1 cm to improve detection of dysplasia and cancer.

secondary peristalsis: Organized contractions of the esophagus triggered by distention of the esophageal lumen by food bolus ingestion or by gastroesophageal reflux. This is in contrast to primary peristalsis, which occurs as a reflex to the act of deglutition or eating; *see also* primary peristalsis.

secretin: A hormone produced by S-cells in the proximal small intestine whose role includes stimulation of pancreatic bicarbonate and enzyme release in response to low duodenal pH.

secretin stimulation test: A diagnostic medical test used to assess pancreatic function by measuring secretion of digestive enzymes. After a 12-hour fast, a nasoduodenal tube is placed and a basal level of lipase, amylase, and trypsin is collected. Next, a patient is given a dose of intravenous secretin. Over the next 1 to 2 hours, the pancreatic secretions are measured via aspiration from the nasoduodenal tube. A similar test can be performed to measure serum gastrin in patients suspected to have a gastrin-secreting tumor.

segmental colitis: Chronic mucosal inflammation of a segment of colon located in an area where diverticulosis is present and may mimic IBD. Treatment is with anti-inflammatory medications, such as 5-aminosalicylic acid derivatives, and surgery is effective in severe cases with a low risk of recurrence; *also referred to as* diverticular-associated colitis.

selective internal radiation (SIR) spheres: An oncologic treatment known as SIR-containing microspheres that are delivered to a tumor via a selective arterial branch, where the radiation can target and kill the cancerous cells. It is commonly used for liver metastases from colon cancer and occasionally for hepatocellular carcinoma.

selenium: A chemical element/trace mineral that functions as a cofactor for many enzymatic reactions in the body. Toxicity is rare, but exposure can lead to cirrhosis and GI discomfort. Deficiency may be a complication of gastric bypass surgery, chronic total parenteral nutrition without supplementation, or severe IBD and may present with congestive heart failure, fatigue, hypothyroidism, and mental status changes.

sensitivity: A statistical concept that describes the ability of a test to correctly identify true positives for disease. For example, a test that correctly identifies all patients who have a disease would be a highly sensitive test. In mathematical terms, sensitivity = number of true positives/(number of true positives + number of false negatives).

septal fibrosis: One of the histologic stages in the progression of chronic liver injury to cirrhosis characterized by the development of fibrous connective tissue in the periportal areas forming bridges connecting one periportal area to another without distorting the anatomy of the liver. It is categorized as stage 3 of a possible 4 stages in the Ludwig-Batts scoring system; *also called* bridging fibrosis.

serosa: The outermost membranous layer of numerous body structures and organs, including the intestine, colon, and peritoneal cavity. The serosa is typically a thin membrane that can secrete materials to decrease friction between two adjacent body structures. The esophagus lacks a serosal layer and instead is outlined by adventitia.

serous cystadenoma: An usually benign cystic lesion of the pancreas primarily affecting women in the seventh decade of life that is often found incidentally during cross-sectional imaging. EUS is helpful in making the diagnosis, and the lesion characteristically has a low fluid amylase and low CEA level on cyst fluid analysis. Unless symptomatic, these lesions are usually monitored clinically.

serrated adenoma: Type of colon polyp that has hyperplastic features with increased malignant potential compared with hyperplastic polyps or sessile serrated adenomas. Histologically, serrated crypts and cytologic atypia are frequent findings; *also called* traditional serrated adenoma.

serum ascites albumin gradient: Calculated by subtracting the ascites albumin level from the serum albumin level and can be used to help determine the etiology of ascites. A gradient greater than 1.1 is highly predictive of portal hypertension/liver disease as the inciting factor for the ascites. A gradient less than 1.1 is often indicative of cancer, tuberculosis, or other cause of noncirrhotic ascites.

serum glutamic oxaloacetic transaminase: *Another term for* aspartate aminotransferase.

serum glutamic pyruvic transaminase (SGPT): *Another term for* alanine aminotransferase.

sessile: Nomenclature used to describe a polyp that is flat (ie, not raised from the mucosa or existing on a stalk).

sessile serrated adenoma: A type of colon polyp usually located in the right colon or cecum that is considered premalignant through a genetic pathway other than the APC pathway that accounts for traditional adenomatous polyps. Histologically, basal crypt dilation is common, but they lack nuclear changes; *also called* sessile serrated polyp.

sessile serrated polyp: *Another term for* sessile serrated adenoma.

Shiga-like toxin: A toxin produced by certain *E coli* strains that damages the vascular endothelium, causing hemorrhage and bloody diarrhea and could result in kidney failure/hemolytic uremic syndrome.

Shigella: A gram-negative bacterial infection that is a common cause of infectious colitis, presenting as abdominal pain and diarrhea with or without bleeding. It is spread via fecal-oral contamination and may be acquired from food contamination. Frequent hand washing and proper disposal of dirty diapers and soiled items can decrease the likelihood of transmission. The typical course of infection and symptoms is 5 to 7 days. Treatment is not required for most cases, but in patients who are immunocompromised or severe cases (such as those with bloody diarrhea), treatment with antibiotics, such as a fluoro-quinolone, is indicated.

shock liver: *See* ischemic hepatopathy.

short bowel syndrome: A severe form of maldigestion in which inadequate nutrients and minerals are absorbed by the intestine, potentially leading to nutritional deficiencies and death. It usually occurs after resection of more than half of the bowel (eg, after necrotizing enterocolitis in children or with Crohn's disease and multiple surgeries in adults). Treatment includes oral rehydrating solutions and parenteral nutrition and may even include intestinal transplantation. Intestinal adaptation may occur, allowing some patients to be converted back to all-oral nutrition.

short-segment Barrett's esophagus: An area of intestinal metaplasia consistent with Barrett's esophagus that extends less than 3 cm in length from the gastroesophageal junction.

short-segment Hirschsprung's disease: A variant of Hirschsprung's disease in which the aganglionic segments are limited to the rectosigmoid colon only. Management is similar to Hirschsprung's disease and usually requires surgery with anorectal myomectomy.

Shwachman-Bodian-Diamond syndrome: *Another term for* Shwachman's syndrome.

Shwachman-Diamond syndrome: *Another term for* Shwachman's syndrome.

Shwachman's syndrome: A rare congenital autosomal recessive disorder characterized by pancreatic insufficiency, low blood counts, and growth deficiency. The pancreatic insufficiency, which usually improves as patients age, may be detected by the presence of steatorrhea, impaired digestion, or growth retardation. Pancreatic enzyme supplementation is often required, but the blood count abnormalities predispose patients to infections and malignancies; *also called* Shwachman-Diamond syndrome, Shwachman-Bodian-Diamond syndrome.

sicca syndrome: The association of dry eyes and dry mouth, in the absence of the arthritis and serum markers found in Sjögren's syndrome. Sicca syndrome symptoms may accompany primary biliary cirrhosis or other chronic liver diseases.

sigmoid colon: A section of large bowel that is located between the descending colon and the rectum. It is a common site of diverticulosis and colon polyps that is easily accessible by sigmoidoscopy or colonoscopy.

sigmoidoscopy: An endoscopic procedure where a thin scope is passed through the rectum into the large bowel to visually inspect the lumen of the sigmoid colon and rectum. The most proximal point the scope can intubate is usually the distal transverse colon. Its primary indications are CRC screening and evaluation of lower GI bleeding. It has largely been replaced by colonoscopy for CRC screening because it examines less than half of the colon; however, it is a better alternative to no screening in regions where colonoscopy is not routinely available. Biopsies can be taken through the scope, and polyps can be removed during the procedure.

sigmoid volvulus: An acute condition that occurs when a segment of the sigmoid colon hinges and twists on itself. Due to its anatomic ability to be somewhat mobilized, the sigmoid colon is the section of bowel most often involved in a volvulus. Volvulus may lead to interruption of the blood supply to the sigmoid and cause ischemia; thus, it carries a risk of perforation and death. Colonoscopic decompression or surgical correction is often urgently necessary.

single balloon enteroscopy: An endoscopic technique used to examine distal portions of the small intestine outside the reach of a standard upper endoscope or push enteroscopy. It uses an endoscope fitted with an overtube that has an inflating balloon at its tip. After the endoscope is advanced forward, the balloon is inflated and the endoscope is pulled backward, producing a pleating effect on the more proximal intestine, decreasing the length the endoscope must travel, and allowing for deeper visualization.

sinusoidal obstruction syndrome: *Another term for* veno-occlusive disease.

Sister Mary Joseph nodule: A palpable lymph node in the periumbilical area that is associated with metastatic intra-abdominal or pelvic cancer, particularly gastric cancer. It is named for the surgical assistant who first appreciated the examination finding.

Sjögren's syndrome: An autoimmune disease characterized by inflammation of the exocrine salivary and lacrimal glands causing dry mouth and dry eyes. It can occur independently or as a systemic disease involving the skin, nose, joints, and vagina. It can also occur in association with other autoimmune diseases, specifically primary biliary cirrhosis or autoimmune hepatitis. Anti-SS-A (Ro) and SS-B (La) antibodies are usually present.

sleeve gastrectomy: A form of weight loss surgery in which 75% of the stomach is removed to reduce the size and capacity of the stomach, leading to weight loss via restriction of oral intake and early satiety. The remnant stomach resembles a sleeve, hence its name. The procedure leaves the biliary anatomy in its anatomical position. It can be performed either open or laparoscopically.

sliding hiatal hernia: Movement of the proximal stomach through the esophageal hiatus in the diaphragm that can predispose individuals to gastroesophageal reflux, esophagitis, and dyspepsia. Incarceration rarely occurs, and surgery is not recommended for this condition. It can be diagnosed by barium esophagram or endoscopy. Treatment is aimed at associated symptoms.

slow transit constipation: A functional disorder of decreased bowel movements due to delayed transit through the colon despite normal-appearing lumen. It is thought to occur in approximately 15% to 30% of patients with chronic constipation. Therapy consists of a high-fiber diet, laxatives, and motility agents as the first few steps. If no relief occurs with those options, sacral nerve stimulation, biofeedback, and surgery may be indicated. It can be diagnosed using a colonic transit test; *also called* colonic inertia.

small bowel bacterial overgrowth: A disorder of increased bacterial expansion in the small intestine leading to symptoms of bloating, diarrhea, dyspepsia, and vitamin B.

selective internal radiation (SIR) spheres: An oncologic treatment known as SIR-containing microspheres that are delivered to a tumor via a selective arterial branch, where the radiation can target and kill the cancerous cells. It is commonly used for liver metastases from colon cancer and occasionally for hepatocellular carcinoma deficiency as a result of malabsorption. It most often occurs in an area of stasis within the small bowel, triggered by decreased motility from autonomic dysfunction (eg, diabetes mellitus), intermittent bowel obstruction, or anatomic variation postoperatively. It is most easily diagnosed with breath testing and can be treated with antibiotics, although several courses of antibiotics may be necessary if the underlying condition is not improved. The traditional standard for diagnosis is jejunal aspirate, although it is uncommonly performed.

small bowel biopsy: Removal of a piece of small intestine for pathologic interpretation. This is most easily achieved using biopsy forceps through an endoscope during an upper endoscopy or colonoscopy. Surgical full-thickness biopsies of the small bowel may be used in the diagnostic workup of suspected Crohn's disease.

small bowel follow through: A radiological procedure in which oral contrast is ingested and serial images of the abdomen are taken over a period of several hours in an effort to evaluate the small intestine for IBD, strictures, tumors, or ulceration.

small intestine: The portion of the GI tract connecting the stomach to the large intestine. It is made up of 3 major segments—the duodenum, jejunum, and ileum—and is referred to as the small bowel. It is the major site of nutrient absorption and a rare site of GI bleeding or malignancy.

SMART pill: A wireless, single-use, digestible device, roughly the size of a multivitamin tablet, used in the evaluation of GI motility disorders. Sensors inside the device can measure pH, pressure, and temperature and that information can be downloaded wirelessly, allowing for rapid interpretation.

snare: An endoscopic tool used during colonoscopy or sigmoidoscopy to remove polyps that can be used with or without cautery. As a verb, it refers to the ability to remove a polyp using the snare tool.

snare cautery polypectomy: Removal of a polyp during a sigmoidoscopy or colonoscopy using a combination of an endoscopic snare and electrocautery. This is the standard technique to remove polyps larger than 6 mm that are encountered during a colonoscopy, especially those that are pedunculated.

solid pseudopapillary neoplasm: A rare, usually benign tumor of the pancreas almost exclusively discovered in young women either incidentally or after presentation with abdominal pain. EUS can be helpful in making the diagnosis by finding an isoechoic or hypoechoic mass with sheets or nests of cells on cytologic evaluation of fine-needle aspiration. Surgery is the treatment of choice because the neoplasm does have a small risk of malignancy, although the operation varies depending on the location of the tumor.

solitary rectal ulcer syndrome: A rare disorder of the rectum in which patients may experience rectal bleeding, rectal pain, abdominal pain, constipation, or diarrhea that is diagnosed by biopsy findings of fibromuscular obliteration and crypt distortion. Despite its name, patients may have more than one lesion and can present without ulcers. However, ulcers are the most common endoscopic finding and are usually located on the anterior rectal wall approximately 10 cm from the anal verge. Treatment may include dietary modification to include more fiber and water, topical anti-inflammatory medications, biofeedback, or surgery.

somatostatin: An inhibitory protein hormone secreted by D-cells in the upper GI tract and pancreas whose effects include slowing the GI system by decreasing blood flow and gastric emptying time, as well as inhibiting the release of pancreatic enzymes.

somatostatinoma: A rare and potentially malignant tumor of the somatostatin-producing D cells in the pancreas or GI tract leading to overproduction of the hormone that can lead to diabetes mellitus, steatorrhea, gallstones, and increased gastric acidity. Most patients present with metastatic disease at the time of diagnosis.

somatostatin-receptor scintigraphy: A radiological test using radioactively labeled octreotide that, when injected intravenously, will bind to tumor cells possessing somatostain receptors and can be used for localizing neuroendocrine cancers; *also called* an Octreoscan.

Sonde enteroscopy: A type of small intestinal endoscopy that uses an endoscope with a balloon at its tip that when inflated is pulled through the small bowel by peristalsis. Mucosal examination is then performed on withdrawal of the scope. It is a mechanism to examine the entire small intestine. Because this procedure routinely takes more than 3 hours to perform, it has largely been replaced by newer techniques to evaluate the small intestine, such as wireless capsule endoscopy and device-assisted enteroscopy.

spastic pelvic floor syndrome: *Another term for* anismus.

specificity: A statistical concept that describes the ability of a test to accurately identify true negatives. For example, a test that correctly identifies all patients who do not have a disease would be a highly specific test. In mathematical terms, specificity = number of true negatives/(number of true negatives + number of false positives).

sphincter of Oddi dysfunction: A motility disorder of the muscular sphincter controlling the outlet of the biliary and pancreatic ducts leading to chronic abdominal pain and possibly to liver enzyme test elevations, usually occurring only in patients who are post-cholecystectomy. The diagnosis is usually based on sphincter manometry and treatment includes anti-spasmodics, plus endoscopic or surgical sphincterotomy; *see* Appendix 25.

sphincterotomy: Surgical or endoscopic opening of the sphincter of Oddi. It is often performed to enable biliary procedures, such as balloon extraction or stent placement, or as a treatment for sphincter of Oddi dysfunction.

spider angioma: A cutaneous finding in which a tuft of small dilated blood vessels radiates outward from a center spot, reminiscent of a spider. Although often benign, such as in pregnancy, it can be a sign of liver disease and portal hypertension.

spiral enteroscopy: A type of device-assisted enteroscopy using a specialized overtube for an enteroscope with a rotating corkscrew mechanism to pleat the intestine over the scope to shorten the length of the intestine and propel the scope forward. It is most often used in the evaluation of obscure GI bleeding or in patients with a positive wireless capsule endoscopy study.

spleen: The anatomic organ located under the left side of the diaphragm whose primary roles include blood filtration and immune function via the reticuloendothelial system and protection against encapsulated bacterial infection.

splenic flexure: The section of colon located at the junction of the descending and transverse colons that, in situ, is typically near the spleen.

splenic vein thrombosis: Acute or chronic obstruction of the main drainage vessel of the spleen by clot. It can occur due to chronic pancreatitis, pancreatic cancer in the tail of the pancreas, hypercoagulable states, or as a result of trauma. Gastric varices may form in patients with splenic vein thrombosis. Treatment is indicated only in patients who are symptomatic, such as those with bleeding gastric varices, and splenectomy is the main treatment.

splenomegaly: An enlarged spleen, most commonly as a consequence of portal hypertension or splenic vein thrombosis. Thrombocytopenia often occurs in patients with splenomegaly due to splenic sequestration of platelets.

spontaneous bacterial peritonitis (SBP): A complication of cirrhosis in which ascitic fluid becomes spontaneously infected, causing abdominal pain, fevers, or both, although it can also present without any symptoms other than abdominal distention with ascites. The diagnosis is made by paracentesis fluid analysis showing an absolute neutrophil count greater than 250, a positive fluid bacterial culture, or both. Treatment is with a third-generation cephalosporin or fluoroquinolone and intravenous albumin. The presence of SBP is a poor prognostic indicator in a patient with cirrhosis and should prompt his or her provider to refer the patient for liver transplant evaluation. It is thought to occur via bacterial translocation from the GI tract into the protein-deficient environment of ascites that cannot defend the bacterial introduction leading to infection.

squamocolumnar junction: The area where the stomach and esophagus meet and the squamous epithelium of the esophagus transitions into the columnar epithelium of the stomach. It is usually located approximately 40 cm from the incisors, as measured during an endoscopy, and is the most common site of Barrett's esophagus and reflux esophagitis.

squamous: A type of epithelial lining found on the skin, as well as in the esophagus and anus within the GI tract.

squamous cell carcinoma: Cancer arising from squamous epithelium. The most common site of squamous cell carcinoma is the skin, where it has low metastatic potential; however, it can also arise in the lung, esophagus, head and neck, and genitourinary tract. Treatment varies depending on the primary site. Esophageal squamous cell carcinoma is the most common form of esophageal cancer outside of the United States, whereas esophageal adenocarcinoma is more common in the United States.

status post: A phrase often used in medicine to refer to a previous intervention (eg, a person who has had his or her appendix removed is status post appendectomy).

steatohepatitis: Inflammation in the liver secondary to fat that can be caused by alcohol or by NAFLD typically associated with components of the metabolic syndrome. Its severity is evaluated using the NAFLD Activity Score. It is a leading cause of what was previously considered cryptogenic cirrhosis in the United States and is a common indication for liver transplantation if end-stage liver disease develops.

steatorrhea: A term used to describe stool with a higher than usual fat component, often causing the stool to float in the toilet water rather than sink. It may also appear to have oily droplets in the toilet water. Its presence suggests fat malabsorption in the intestinal tract and is often a sign of pancreatic insufficiency. Stool can be tested in a laboratory for fecal fat qualitatively or quantitatively to help make the diagnosis.

stellate scar: A radiographic finding in the liver on computed tomography described as a lesion with a hypoattenuating central area and radiating fibrous septa. It is present in up to one-third of focal nodular hyperplasia cases.

stent: A small tube inserted into an anatomic area to treat a narrowing/stricture, prevent blockages from occurring, or maintain patency of a structure. Stents can be made of plastic or metallic material and can be coated or uncoated with various chemicals. They are often used in the management of biliary strictures, pancreatic duct strictures, and malignant strictures from esophageal or colon cancer.

stercoral ulcer: Mucosal erosion that forms in the distal colon or rectum as a result of severe constipation and subsequent irritation of the mucosal lining. Symptoms include rectal pain, lower GI bleeding, and, rarely, perforation. Treatment includes stool softeners, endoscopic control of hemorrhage, and surgery if perforation occurs.

sterile pancreatic necrosis: Nonviable, uninfected dead pancreatic tissue, usually as a result of severe acute pancreatitis. Over time, this type of tissue can wall off and form a fluid collection leading to pain, biliary obstruction, nausea, vomiting, weight loss, and infection. It is usually recommended that the pancreatic necrotic tissue be debrided once it has walled off, and debridement can be performed endoscopically, percutaneously, or surgically.

Stevens-Johnson syndrome: A potentially life-threatening dermatologic condition of skin desquamation and severe mucosal ulceration often triggered by a medication hypersensitivity reaction or infection. In hepatology, it should be recognized as a rare complication of telaprevir-based antiviral therapy for hepatitis C.

stigmata of recent bleeding: Endoscopic findings in the GI tract, such as adherent clot, visible vessels, or red wale, seen after a GI bleed that are helpful in determining the source of bleeding, as well as predicting the risk of rebleeding. They are one of the components of the Rockall score.

stomach: A muscular anatomic structure located in the abdomen that receives ingested food from the esophagus and initiates the process of digestion before passing the food into the duodenum through the pylorus. Digestion phases occurring in the stomach include temporary food storage, mechanical food breakdown, and gastric acid and enzymatic exposure. Many hormones and other molecules involved in digestion, including pepsinogen, gastrin, and intrinsic factor, are also created in the stomach.

stool: Another name for human feces, the waste product of digestion, that is dispelled from the colon through bowel movements. Regular stool frequency ranges from 3 times per week to 3 times per day.

stool chymotrypsin activity: A commercially available stool biochemical test used to indirectly assess exocrine pancreatic function. Lower levels of the enzymatic activity of chymotrypsin in the stool are consistent with chronic pancreatitis.

stool osmotic gap: The difference between measured and calculated stool osmolality, where calculated stool osmolality is derived from 2 times the sum of sodium and potassium ions in the stool. This test can be used to differentiate between osmotic and secretory diarrhea. In osmotic diarrhea (eg, laxative abuse or after a colonoscopy prep), an unmeasured substance exists and creates an osmotic gap larger than 50 to 100 mOsm/kg. The gap is smaller than 50 mOsm/kg in patients with secretory diarrhea.

stool pH: A measurement of the acid/base status of stool used in the diagnosis of chronic diarrhea. The normal range is 7.0 to 7.5. A stool pH level less than 5.5 is consistent with a carbohydrate absorption abnormality and can cause perianal erythema and excoriation. Alkaline pH can be seen with secretory diarrheas and IBD/colitis and in diarrhea associated with large villous adenomas.

stricture: A narrowing of the GI tract that can occur anywhere from the esophagus to the anus, causing obstruction of the flow of luminal contents. Acid exposure is a common cause of peptic strictures in the esophagus and IBD is often associated with strictures, commonly in the terminal ileum. Medications that treat excess acid or IBD may also reverse a mild stricture, but endoscopic dilatation or surgical intervention is usually required in the management of chronic strictures.

Strongyloides stercoralis: A parasitic nematode that causes the disease strongyloidiasis, most commonly seen in tropical areas. The infection can cause dermatologic changes (such as urticarial), pulmonary distress (Loffler's syndrome), and disseminated infection, particularly in patients who are immunocompromised. Disseminated disease can present with abdominal pain, abdominal distention, and signs of shock. Ivermectin and albendazole are used for treatment.

subepithelial: The layers of the GI tract just below the mucosa. This term is used to describe lesions or masses that do not break the mucosal lining but are prominently protruding into the lumen of the GI tract. Standard biopsies may not be able to obtain tissue from this layer and other imaging modalities may be required.

subepithelial mass: A growth originating from beneath the mucosa of the GI tract. These are often noticed incidentally on endoscopy and may require additional testing, such as endoscopic ultrasonography with or without fine-needle aspiration or CT scan to aid in the diagnosis.

submucosal: Located beneath the mucosa of the GI tract; *also referred to as* subepithelial, although submucosal refers to the more specific layer just beneath the mucosa called the *submucosa* and does not typically include the muscular layers. Masses such as lipomas and GI stromal tumors often arise from this layer.

superior mesenteric artery: A major arterial branch of the aorta located just below the celiac trunk that typically supplies blood flow to the small and large intestine, as well as the pancreas. Thrombosis of this artery can cause abdominal pain and intestinal ischemia.

superior mesenteric artery syndrome: A rare condition in which the third portion of the duodenum is trapped between the aorta and the superior mesenteric artery. The typical presentation is of chronic intermittent abdominal pain associated with episodic vomiting, nausea, and occasional bowel obstruction. It can also present acutely after scoliosis surgery or after rapid weight loss, both of which act to change the aortomesenteric angle predisposing to the condition. Treatment is aimed at reversing precipitating factors and may include enteral or parenteral nutrition or surgical intervention.

survival analysis: A statistical method used to study longitudinal data on the time until the occurrence of the event of interest. For example, this method can be used to predict how long it would take to develop recurrent colon cancer after surgical resection.

sustained virologic response: Undetectable virus in the blood of a patient treated for hepatitis C at 24 weeks after therapy completion. Originally, this term referred to normalization of liver enzymes persisting 24 weeks after completion of interferon-based therapy for hepatitis C. It is thought of by many as a marker of hepatitis C cure. This term can also be used to refer to shorter periods of time after treatment completion by designating the week number after SVR (eg, SVR12 = sustained virologic response 12 weeks after treatment completion).

swallow-induced peristalsis: *Another term for* primary peristalsis.

synchronous: The coexistence of 2 events or conditions. In gastroenterology, this term is most frequently used to describe the presence of 2 separate colon cancers diagnosed at the same time or within 6 months of original diagnosis.

systemic sclerosis: An autoimmune disorder characterized by collagen deposition in the skin and organs, including the esophagus and small bowel. It most commonly affects young women. GI effects of this illness include gastroesophageal reflux, dysphagia, constipation, and small intestinal bacterial overgrowth.

Terry's nails: The name for a specific change in the color and appearance of the nails, in which the majority of the nail turns white and the distal aspect of the nail may be darker or reddened. Initially described in patients with cirrhosis, it has also been seen in those with other chronic conditions, such as diabetes mellitus or chronic congestive heart failure.

tetrahydrocannabinol (THC) receptor: *Another term for* cannabinoid receptor.

thiamine: A B-complex vitamin, *also known as* vitamin B_1, which plays an essential role in numerous aspects of metabolism and nervous system function. It is obtained solely from the diet and is absorbed in the small intestine. Deficiency, common in alcoholics, results in damage to the heart and nervous system, known as beriberi.

thiopurine methyltransferase (TPMT): An enzyme that is responsible for metabolizing thiopurine compounds, which are found in several pharmacologic drugs, such as azathioprine, 6-mercaptopurine, and thioguanine. Genetic variations can cause a decrease in the activity of this enzyme, and in affected individuals this may result in severe toxicity if treated with thiopurine medications. The level of TPMT activity can be measured by a blood test and used to individualize dosing with drugs containing thiopurine compounds; *see* Appendix 14.

thrombocytopenia: A decrease in the circulating number of platelets in the bloodstream due to decreased production, sequestration, or increased platelet destruction. Portal hypertension may result in splenomegaly and platelet sequestration in the spleen, resulting in thrombocytopenia. Viruses, such as hepatitis C, can also be associated with immune thrombocytopenic purpura, an autoimmune destruction of platelets.

tissue transglutaminase IgA, IgG: Autoantibodies that form against the enzyme tissue transglutaminase (tTG), which is the major autoantigen in celiac disease. The test for tTG-IgA antibodies is very sensitive and specific for the diagnosis of small bowel injury in patients with celiac disease who are exposed to gluten. In patients with IgA deficiency, testing for IgG antibodies is more diagnostic because IgA antibodies may be falsely negative.

total parenteral nutrition (TPN): The provision of calories, vitamins, and minerals via intravenous infusion, bypassing the intestinal tract. This requires central venous access for delivery and carries an increased risk of fungal infections and bacteremia compared with enteral nutrition.

Toupet procedure: A surgical procedure performed to treat gastroesophageal reflux disease in which the fundus is wrapped around the posterior aspect of the esophagus to reinforce an incompetent lower esophageal sphincter and prevent acid from refluxing back into the esophagus.

toxic megacolon: An acute, severe form of colonic inflammation associated with *C difficile* infection, IBD, cytomegalovirus, and other forms of infectious colitis. It is defined by a radiographically dilated colon (larger than 6 cm in the transverse colon) and evidence of severe infection evidenced by three of four criteria—fever, tachycardia, leukocytosis, or anemia—and at least one of the following signs or symptoms: dehydration, change in mental status, serious electrolyte deviation, or hypotension. Prompt surgical consultation is imperative in management because many patients require colectomy. Intravenous steroids and anti-tumor necrosis factor agents may also be helpful in IBD-related disease.

trachealization of the esophagus: The development of circumferential rings inside the lumen of the esophagus, resembling those of the trachea, as seen during endoscopic evaluation in patients with eosinophilic esophagitis; *also known as* feline esophagus.

tracheoesophageal fistula: An anomalous connection between the trachea and the esophagus that can be congenital or acquired later in life. Some acquired causes include esophageal cancer and tracheal injury that occurs during prolonged mechanical intubation.

traditional serrated adenoma: *Another term for* serrated adenoma.

transgastric peritoneoscopy: A form of NOTES, a novel technique used to gain access to the peritoneal cavity. An endoscope is inserted through the mouth, down the esophagus, and into the stomach where an incision is made through the wall of the stomach to gain access to the peritoneal cavity for diagnostic and potentially therapeutic purposes.

transient lower esophageal sphincter relaxation: Episodic reduction in basal intraluminal pressure within the lower esophageal sphincter. This occurs physiologically during a swallow, but frequent and excessive episodes may be associated with pathologic gastroesophageal reflux.

transjugular: Across or through the jugular vein, which is often used as a point of entry into the venous system for various types of interventional procedures, including right heart catheterization, liver pressure measurements, and liver biopsy.

transjugular intrahepatic portosystemic shunt (TIPS): A procedure performed by an interventional radiologist in which a connection is created between a branch of the hepatic vein and a branch of the portal vein for the purpose of decreasing portal pressure in patients with portal hypertension. Indications for TIPS include refractory ascites or hydrothorax in the setting of cirrhosis and variceal hemorrhage unable to be controlled endoscopically. Possible complications include hepatic encephalopathy, right-sided heart failure, progressive liver dysfunction, occlusion of the artificial connection by blood clot or stenosis, infection, and bleeding. The MELD score was originally designed to predict mortality after TIPS, with a MELD score greater than 18 predicting significant risk.

transjugular liver biopsy: Acquisition of liver tissue using a transjugular approach. A thin catheter is inserted into the jugular vein and threaded through the vena cava and into the right hepatic vein. A special type of needle is then guided over the catheter and into a section of the liver to procure a tissue sample. This is the preferred method of liver biopsy in patients with a bleeding diathesis or those who cannot undergo a percutaneous biopsy, such as in patients with ascites or abdominal wall cellulitis.

transmural: Across the full-thickness of the wall of an organ. For example, Crohn's disease is characterized by transmural inflammation of the small bowel or colon.

transmural drainage: An endoscopic therapy often used to treat pancreatic pseudocysts by which the endoscopist creates a connection between a cyst and the GI lumen by extending all the way across the GI wall to decompress the cyst.

transpapillary: Across or extending through the duodenal papilla (at the ampulla of Vater).

transpapillary drainage: An endoscopic procedure used to promote drainage of bile, pancreatic secretions, or peripancreatic fluid collections by using therapeutic instruments across the duodenal papilla (at the ampulla of Vater).

transplant: The act of removing tissue or an organ from the body of a donor and placing it in the body of a recipient. In an autologous transplant, the donor and recipient are the same person. In an allogenic transplant, the donor and recipient are two genetically nonidentical individuals. Within gastroenterology, successful transplantation is frequently performed in liver, small bowel, and pancreas.

transplant hepatology: An American Board of Internal Medicine–recognized subspecialty within the field of gastroenterology that focuses on the perioperative and long-term care of patients with acute or chronic liver disease, during all phases of liver transplantation.

transplant surgery: A surgical subspecialty focused on transplanting organs from donors to recipients. Transplant surgeons are involved in the procurement of donor organs and the implantation of the organ into the recipient.

transsinusoidal pressure gradient: The difference in pressure between the portal vein and the hepatic vein across the liver sinusoids, as measured during a transjugular study. This is often elevated in patients with cirrhosis and portal hypertension. A gradient higher than 6 mm Hg is consistent with portal hypertension and a gradient between 10 and 12 mm Hg predicts increased risk of forming varices and ascites.

transverse colon: Portion of the colon that extends between the hepatic and splenic flexures, typically coursing transversely across the upper abdomen.

trichrome stain: A staining technique commonly used in pathology that produces three colors to distinguish between different parts of a cell. Nuclei are stained blue, collagen is usually green (or may be blue depending on technique), and cytoplasm is bright red. It is often used to highlight fibrous connective tissue, especially in liver biopsies.

trimbath syndrome: A subset of Lynch syndrome in which patients have specific genetic mutations of one of four mismatch repair genes. Patients may present with café au lait spots, lymphoma, extracolonic tumors including glioblastoma, and CRC at a young age.

tropical sprue: A malabsorptive disease of the small intestine that most often occurs in those visiting or living in the tropics. It usually manifests as malabsorption after an acute diarrheal infection. Treatment is with antibiotics for 3 to 6 months and vitamin supplementation.

Trousseau's syndrome: The development of a blood clot or clots anywhere in the body associated with an occult malignancy. Armand Trousseau originally described it in 1865 and then, coincidentally, later diagnosed himself with and died of gastric cancer.

Truelove and Witts' classification: A set of criteria created to define the severity of ulcerative colitis. The severity may be defined as mild, moderate, or severe based on the number of bloody stools per day, temperature, heart rate, hemoglobin, and erythrocyte sedimentation rate. Classification may aid in the decision making regarding treatment or be useful for evaluation of an investigational therapy's effect on ulcerative colitis. It is named for British gastroenterologists Drs. SC Truelove and Leslie Witts.

trypsin: A digestive enzyme produced by the pancreas that breaks down proteins into their individual amino acids.

trypsinogen: The inactive form of trypsin, produced by the pancreas. This enzyme requires breakdown into its active form—trypsin—to function in its role in protein digestion.

TTS: An abbreviation for "through the scope," typically referring to balloon dilation through an endoscope to treat a stricture or any other lesion compromising luminal diameter and flow.

t-tube: A hollow T-shaped tube placed surgically oriented so that the two short limbs are in the bile duct and the long limb drains externally. It is often used to maintain patency of the bile duct and effective bile drainage following surgical procedures on the bile duct, including liver transplantation.

tubular adenoma: A neoplasm of colonic or intestinal epithelium with cells more crowded and glands more elongated than normal mucosa but still arranged in a recognizable tubular pattern. This is the most common type of colon polyp; *see also* adenomatous polyp.

tubulovillous adenoma: A neoplasm of colonic or intestinal epithelium that contains features of tubular adenoma with cells arranged in a tubular pattern, as well as features of villous adenoma with cells arranged in a pattern of elongated glandular structures with a cauliflower-like appearance. In the colon polyp to cancer sequence, it is thought to be an intermediary stage between an early neoplasm (tubular adenoma) and more advanced neoplasm (villous adenoma).

Turcot's syndrome: *See* Crail's syndrome.

tylosis: An autosomal dominant genetic condition characterized by thickening, or hyperkeratosis, of the palms and soles. It is associated with the development of squamous cell carcinoma of the esophagus.

Type V choledochal cyst: *Another term for* Caroli's disease.

typhlitis: An enterocolitis affecting the ileocecal region in a patient with neutropenia, most often due to chemotherapy. The inflammation commonly results in necrosis of the bowel wall and can be life threatening. It usually resolves once neutropenia recovers.

ulcerative colitis: An idiopathic inflammatory disease of the mucosal layer of the colon. The rectum is always involved, and continuous inflammation may extend proximally throughout the colon. Patients present with bloody diarrhea, abdominal pain, fatigue, and fevers. Extraintestinal involvement can occur, including articular, ocular, and dermatologic complications. Diagnosis is confirmed with colonoscopy and biopsy. Treatment includes anti-inflammatory agents, corticosteroids, immunomodulators, and surgery; *see* Appendix 16.

ulcerative jejunitis: A rare complication of celiac disease with multiple chronic ulcers throughout the jejunum. Patients respond poorly to a gluten-free diet and steroids, and mortality approaches 30%. It is thought to be a precursor to intestinal T-cell lymphoma.

ultrashort-segment Hirschsprung's disease: A variant of Hirschsprung's disease causing chronic constipation in the first year of life. Failure of the internal anal sphincter to relax on manometry is required for diagnosis. In contrast to classic Hirschsprung's disease, there may be ganglion cells on rectal biopsy, and there is no transition zone seen on barium enema. Treatment consists of anorectal myomectomy, in which a strip of muscle near the anus is removed.

umbilical hernia: Defect in the anterior abdominal wall at the umblicus. This condition can be congenital in children, whereas adults usually present with an acquired form secondary to obesity, abdominal surgery, pregnancy, or ascites. Open or laparascopic surgical repair is usually required if symptomatic, and many patients pursue surgery even for cosmetic reasons in the absence of symptoms.

Fenkel JM, ed.
Quick Reference Dictionary for GI and Hepatology (pp 199-200).
© 2014 Taylor & Francis Group.

uncinate process: A projection of the head of the pancreas. This structure passes anterior to the aorta and inferior vena cava and posterior to the superior mesenteric vessels.

upper esophageal sphincter: A complex muscle interaction composed of the proximal portion of the cervical esophagus, the cricopharyngeus muscle, and the inferior pharyngeal constrictor. The upper esophageal sphincter remains closed at rest and relaxes to facilitate swallowing.

upper GI series: *Another term for* a barium swallow.

upper gastrointestinal hemorrhage: Bleeding proximal to the ligament of Treitz. Patients often present with hematemesis of frank blood, coffee-ground emesis, or melena. Hematochezia can occur in the setting of a brisk upper GI hemorrhage. The common differential diagnosis includes peptic ulcer disease, varices, mucosal inflammation, arteriovenous malformations, tumors, esophagitis, and Mallory-Weiss tears. Treatment includes resuscitation with crystalloid and colloid solutions, parenteral proton pump inhibitors, endoscopic identification, and treatment of the source of bleeding.

urea breath test: Noninvasive test for the presence of *H pylori*. The patient drinks a solution of ^{13}C-labeled urea, which is hydrolyzed into carbon dioxide by the urease enzyme of the bacteria and then detected in the patient's breath during a positive test.

uveitis: Inflammation of the middle portion of the eye, including the choroid, ciliary body, and iris. Etiologies include local and systemic inflammatory disorders (including IBD), infection, and drugs.

vagotomy: Resection of segments of the vagal nerve that innervate the stomach. This procedure may be useful in the treatment of severe peptic ulcer disease that has failed medical management.

variceal band ligation (VBL): Endoscopic treatment of esophageal varices where a high-pressure elastic band is placed over a varix, causing tamponade and sclerosis. It is the first-line treatment for acute variceal hemorrhage. VBL can be used to prevent bleeding in newly diagnosed large varices, those with high risk bleeding stigmata, or those who are intolerant or ineligible for nonselective beta-blocker therapy as prophylaxis.

varix/varices: Swollen vein(s) in the GI tract or abdomen that occur as a result of portal hypertension due to cirrhosis and increased transsinusoidal pressure. The most common locations are the esophagus, stomach, and rectum. Varices form at a rate of approximately 7% per year in patients with portal hypertension.

vasoactive intestinal peptide (VIP): A peptide produced in many tissues, including the pancreas, gut, nerve ganglion, and hypothalamus, that stimulates intestinal secretion of electrolytes and water, dilates vascular beds, and relaxes smooth muscle.

veno-occlusive disease: A serious complication of stem cell transplantation and some chemotheraputic agents. The pathogenesis is related to hepatic vascular endothelial injury, sinusoidal obstruction and dilatation, and hepatic necrosis. Presentation classically includes painful hepatomegaly, weight gain, ascites, jaundice, and, in severe cases, death; *also called* sinusoidal obstruction syndrome.

Fenkel JM, ed.
Quick Reference Dictionary for GI and Hepatology (pp 201-205).
© 2014 Taylor & Francis Group.

Verner-Morrison syndrome: *Also termed* pancreatic cholera or WDHA syndrome, this syndrome consists of watery diarrhea, hypokalemia, achlorhydria, and metabolic acidosis. It is associated with the overproduction of VIP from a pancreatic islet cell tumor either in isolation or as part of the multiple endocrine neoplasia syndrome type 1. This syndrome was named for American physicians John Verner and Ashton Morrison, who described the syndrome in 1958.

vertical banded gastroplasty: Open or laparoscopic procedure used for the treatment of morbid obesity. A small pouch is created along the lesser curvature of the stomach to create early satiety and to cause weight loss. This pouch empties through a banded outlet into the remaining stomach. The band can be tightened or loosened to control the size of the pouch and thus the weight loss.

Vibrio: Genus of anaerobic bacteria, many of which cause severe diarrheal illness. Species include *V cholerae* (the causative agent of cholera), *V parahaemolyticus,* and *V vulnificus. Vibrio* can contaminate seafood and seawater. Immunocompromised hosts are more susceptible to severe infection, including sepsis.

vigorous achalasia: Normal or high-amplitude, simultaneous esophageal body contractions against a lower esophageal sphincter with absent relaxation. The disease may progress to classic achalasia (with absent or low-amplitude contractions), and the treatment is identical for both.

villi: Thin, fingerlike projections that line the mucosa of the small intestine to increase the surface area of the bowel for absorption of nutrients.

villous: A histologic term describing a finding that resembles the mucosal lining of the small intestine.

villous adenoma: A type of polyp most commonly found in the rectosigmoid colon with villous histology. Villous adenomas constitute 10% of colonic adenomas and have a significantly higher malignant potential (approximately 25% to 30%) compared with tubular adenomas.

VIPoma: A rare neuroendocrine neoplasm, usually arising in the pancreas, that secretes VIP. It is associated with Verner-Morrison syndrome/pancreatic cholera/WDHA syndrome. The majority of VIPomas have metastasized at the time of diagnosis.

viral esophagitis: Infection of the esophagus with a virus, causing inflammation. Herpes simplex virus is the most common pathogen, whereas other organisms include herpes zoster, HIV, and cytomegalovirus (CMV). It can often present with odynophagia, dysphagia, and chest pain. Most patients are immunocompromised, but infection in immunocompetent hosts can occur. Diagnosis is made with endoscopic biopsies.

viral fitness: The adaptability of a virus to its host environment.

viral gastroenteritis: Inflammation of the stomach and intestines caused by a viral insult, leading to an acute onset of vomiting or diarrhea. RNA viruses, such as norovirus and rotavirus, are common etiologies. The overall infectious course is usually benign and self-limited but can be more severe in young children and the elderly.

viral hepatitis: Inflammation in the liver caused by a viral infection. This term most commonly refers to hepatitis B or C but can also refer to any viral etiology for acute or chronic inflammation.

Virchow's node: A hardened, left, supraclavicular lymph node that is commonly associated with intrabdominal, particularly gastric, malignancy. It is named for 19th century German pathologist Rudolf Virchow.

viscera: Internal organs.

visceral pain: Discomfort originating from an internal organ or its lining. This pain is poorly localizable, dull, often midline, and associated with nausea and other autonomic symptoms. It may be referred to other areas of the body due to convergence of visceral and somatic afferent nerve fibers.

vitamin: A compound necessary for human growth and health that is not synthesized or is inadequately synthesized in the body and thus must be consumed in the diet.

vitamin A (retinol): A fat-soluble vitamin necessary for normal vision, cell growth and differentiation, iron metabolism, and immunity. Deficiency results in immune compromise, night blindness, conjunctival dryness, and keratomalacia (corneal softening). Toxicity, classically from consumption of animal liver, results in dry skin, vomiting, arthralgias, increased cerebral pressure, and rarely liver failure.

vitamin B$_1$ (thiamine): A water-soluble vitamin essential for energy production and peripheral nerve conduction; *see also* thiamine.

vitamin B$_2$ (riboflavin): *See* riboflavin.

vitamin B$_3$: *Another term for* niacin.

vitamin B$_6$ (pyridoxine): A water-soluble vitamin involved in multiple metabolic processes, including amino acid and neurotransmitter synthesis. Deficiency can be due to dietary deficiency, chronic disease, or the effect of certain medications, such as isoniazid. Deficiency results in skin changes, diarrhea, peripheral neuropathy, and personality changes.

vitamin B$_{12}$ (cobalamin): A water-soluble vitamin that requires intrinsic factor for absorption in the terminal ileum and is essential for various metabolic processes, including hematopoiesis and central nervous system function.

vitamin B$_{12}$ deficiency: Deficient levels of vitamin B$_{12}$, which can be caused by inadequate dietary intake, pernicious anemia, small intestinal bacterial overgrowth, or disorders of the pancreas or ileum. Deficiency can manifest with megaloblastic anemia, fatigue, pallor, and smoothing of the tongue. Neurologic symptoms from degeneration of the posterior column of the spinal cord include parasthesias, sensory disturbances, ataxia, and dementia.

vitamin C (ascorbic acid): A water-soluble vitamin involved in a variety of processes, including connective tissue metabolism, iron absorption, and peptide hormone synthesis. Dietary deficiency (scurvy) may cause intra-articular, intrabdominal, and oral bleeding. Excess consumption can result in nausea, vomiting, and diarrhea.

vitamin D: A group of fat-soluble vitamins involved with calcium and phosphorous regulation and bone mineralization. It can be synthesized from steroid precursors by using ultraviolet light exposure from sunlight or can be obtained through the diet. It requires enzymatic conversion in the liver and kidneys into its active form. Vitamin D increases calcium and phosphorous absorption in the intestine and maintains bone mineralization. Deficiency in children (rickets) results in growth retardation and bone abnormalities. Deficiency in adults can result in poorly mineralized, fracture-prone bones (osteomalacia) and is common in patients with chronic liver or kidney disease.

vitamin D 1,25-OH: The active form of vitamin D in the body. It is activated in the kidney by 25-hydroxyvitamin D-1α-hydroxylase.

vitamin D 25-OH: Vitamin D (D3) is converted in the liver by vitamin D-25 hydroxylase into 25-OH vitamin D. The blood level of 25-OH vitamin D is the initial screening test for vitamin D deficiency.

vitamin E: A fat-soluble vitamin required for a variety of metabolic functions, including lipid metabolism. Deficiency occurs only with severe malabsorptive processes and results in axonal degradation with peripheral neuropathy, ataxia, myopathy, and retinopathy. Toxicity can cause impaired coagulation.

vitamin K: A fat-soluble vitamin required for the activation of proteins involved in coagulation. Deficiency can result from poor dietary intake or pathologies of the small bowel that impair absorption or synthesis. Deficiency manifests with impaired coagulation and bleeding.

vitiligo: An autoimmune disorder characterized by depigmented macules, most often on the head, face, mucous membranes, and extremities. It is associated with other autoimmune disorders, including pernicious anemia.

vomiting: The oral expulsion of gastric contents via contraction of gastric, abdominal, and thoracic musculature in response to a noxious stimulus.

Waldmann's disease: *Another term for* primary intestinal lymphangiectasia.

walled-off pancreatic necrosis: A rare, late complication of acute pancreatitis defined as an area of necrosis and infection well-circumscribed by granulation tissue. Treatment involves broad-spectrum antibiotics and percutaneous, endoscopic, or surgical drainage.

Warthin-Starry stain: Silver-nitrate histologic stain used for the visualization of certain bacteria, including *H pylori*, spirochetes, and *B henselae.*

watermelon stomach: *Another name for* gastric antral vascular ectasia.

wedged hepatic venous pressure (WHVP): A transvenously acquired measurement of hepatic sinusoidal pressure using a balloon inflated over a guide wire to estimate the degree of portal venous hypertension and the risk for complications in patients with cirrhosis.

Wernicke-Korsakoff syndrome: A central nervous system disorder in patients with chronic thiamine deficiency, most commonly seen in patients with chronic alcohol abuse. The syndrome is a combination of Wernicke's encephalopathy and Korsakoff psychosis. Treatment is immediate thiamine repletion, but the disease may be irreversible.

Wernicke's encephalopathy: A triad of confusion, ataxia, and ophthalmoplegia (paralysis of the extraocular muscles). It occurs in 1% of alcoholics and is secondary to chronic thiamine deficiency. Immediate parenteral thiamine may reverse the disease, but chronic central nervous system dysfunction is common.

WDHA syndrome: *See* Verner-Morrison syndrome.

Fenkel JM, ed.
Quick Reference Dictionary for GI and Hepatology (pp 206-208)
© 2014 Taylor & Francis Group.

Whipple procedure (pancreaticoduodenectomy): A surgical procedure for the resection of pancreatic head lesions and ampullary masses developed by German surgeon Walther Kausch and perfected by Dr. Allen Whipple. The pancreatic head, distal stomach, duodenum, common bile duct, gallbladder, and proximal jejunum are removed. The stomach, pancreas, and common hepatic ducts are then anastomosed at separate points with the jejunum. Multiple variants exist, including pylorus-preserving pancreaticoduodenectomy.

Whipple's disease: A systemic infection with *Tropheryma Whipplei* that manifests with a classic malabsorbtive wasting syndrome, as well as articular, neurologic, cardiac, and pulmonary involvement. The diagnosis is made via duodenal biopsy revealing Periodic acid-Schiff–positive macrophages. Treatment consists of an extended course of antibiotics.

Whipple's triad: Criteria developed by pancreatic surgeon Allen Whipple to suggest the presence of an insulin-secreting tumor (insulinoma). The triad consists of (1) documentation of hypoglycemia, (2) presence of hypoglycemic symptoms, and (3) resolution of symptoms with administration of glucose.

Wilson's disease: A genetic defect in biliary copper excretion causing copper deposition in the liver and other tissues. Patients from early childhood through the fifth decade of life can present with acute or chronic liver failure, hemolytic anemia, and neuropsychiatric manifestations, such as parkinsonian symptoms, ataxia, and personality changes. Treatment with copper-chelating agents, including d-penicillamine, zinc, and trientine, is effective. Liver transplantation is indicated for severe disease and fulminant hepatic failure; *also called* hepatolenticular degeneration.

wire exchange: An endoscopic technique used to facilitate access to a lumen or cavity. The lumen (eg, a duct or cyst) is cannulated with a guidewire, allowing the operator to deploy instruments and devices over the wire for diagnostic or therapeutic purposes. This is a common technique used during ERCP procedures.

wireless capsule endoscopy: A pill-sized camera that can wirelessly transmit images of the esophagus, stomach, small bowel, and colon. It is most often used in the evaluation of obscure GI bleeding, Crohn's disease, and other small bowel pathologies. Battery life on the camera can last more than 8 hours. The images are recorded on a wireless data recorder that can be easily transferred to a computer for interpretation of the images.

wireless pH monitor: A small recording device that is endoscopically placed near the gastroesophogeal junction and transmits pH measurements wirelessly to an external recorder. It is used to diagnose and assess the severity of GERD and is preferred by patients over traditional intranasal pH monitors for comfort reasons.

xanthelasma palpebra: Cutaneous yellow plaques composed of cholesterol or fat, located around the eyelids. They are a type of xanthoma.

xanthoma: Accumulation of lipid-laden macrophages under the skin associated with familial hypercholesteremias, hyperlipidemia, diabetes mellitus, some malignancies, and primary biliary cirrhosis.

Y90 (Yttrium) spheres: Radioactive spheres used for the treatment of hepatocellular carcinoma. Y90 microspheres are placed by catheter directly into the arteries feeding the tumor. In patients with portal vein thrombosis, it is often preferred over transarterial chemoembolization; *also called* radioembolization, although it is not actually completely embolic as compared with transarterial chemoembolization.

YAG laser (Nd-YAG laser): Neodymium-yttrium-aluminum-garnet laser used for endoscopic tumor ablation and hemostasis in a variety of conditions including radiation proctitis and peptic ulcer disease.

yellow fever: A viral hemorrhagic fever transmitted by mosquitos. Clinical manifestations include fever, myalgias, nausea, and jaundice occurring 3 to 5 days after the infection is acquired. Hepatic necrosis due to microvascular insult is a hallmark of the disease. Severe disease is marked by coagulopathy, renal failure, coma, and death.

Yersinia enterocolitica: A zoonotic bacterium that can cause an acute inflammatory disease of the small intestine and colon, particularly around the terminal ileum. Patients may have terminal ileitis or mesenteric lymphadenopathy that can mimic appendicitis. Individuals with diabetes mellitus and those with iron overload are at highest risk for septicemia.

YMDD sequence: A highly conserved region of the hepatitis B viral DNA polymerase enzyme (Y = tyrosine, M = methionine, D = aspartic acid, D = aspartic acid). Mutations occurring in this region typically confer lamivudine resistance.

Fenkel JM, ed.
Quick Reference Dictionary for GI and Hepatology (pp 210-211).
© 2014 Taylor & Francis Group.

Yueh catheter: Type of needle/catheter system used for removal of fluid from a body cavity. It typically includes a plastic catheter with four side holes introduced by a hollow needle stylet.

Z

Zenker's diverticulum: A pouch-like sac forming near the pharyngoesophageal junction, within Killian's triangle, which can cause dysphagia, halitosis, regurgitation, cough, and aspiration. It is not a true diverticulum and is most common in patients older than 60 years; *also called* pharyngoesophageal diverticulum.

zinc: Atomic element 30; an essential mineral integral to many cellular activities, including wound healing, cell division, DNA and protein synthesis, and immune function. It can also be used as a treatment for Wilson's disease.

zinc deficiency: A syndrome characterized by diarrhea, hair loss, skin lesions (acrodermatitis), anorexia, growth delay, and hypogonadism. It may be caused by inadequate zinc intake (eg, alcoholics, total parenteral nutrition without supplementation) or poor intestinal absorption (eg, Crohn's disease, GI surgery).

Z-line: *See* gastroesophageal junction.

Zollinger-Ellison syndrome (ZE syndrome): A syndrome of hypergastrinemia caused by a gastrin-producing tumor leading to diarrhea, abdominal pain, GI mucosal ulceration, nausea, and vomiting. ZE tumors are most commonly discovered in the pancreatic head or small intestine (gastrinoma triangle) and may be associated with multiple endocrine neoplasia type 1. Proton pump inhibitors are first-line therapy, and surgery is indicated if the tumors are malignant or if symptoms of hypergastrinemia are not controlled by acid suppression.

Fenkel JM, ed.
Quick Reference Dictionary for GI and Hepatology (pp 212).
© 2014 Taylor & Francis Group.

List of Appendices

SECTION I
Liver

Causes of Acute Liver Failure

Acute liver failure is an uncommon disease, and its etiology is best thought of as being infectious, toxin-induced, or host-related. The table below lists the differential diagnosis by category, and then a mnemonic device is provided to help remember the most common causes.

Infectious	Toxin-Induced	Host-Related
Hepatitis A	Acetaminophen	Autoimmune hepatitis
Hepatitis B	Cocaine	Budd-Chiari syndrome
Hepatitis D	Alcoholic hepatitis	Acute fatty liver of pregnancy
Epstein-Barr virus	Mushrooms (*Amanita phylloides*)	Ischemic hepatitis
Herpes simplex virus	Drug-induced liver injury	*Post-liver transplant*
Cytomegalovirus	Herbal/dietary supplement–induced liver injury	Hepatic artery thrombosis
	Carbon tetrachloride	Acute cellular rejection
	Yellow phosphorus	

Fenkel JM, ed.
Quick Reference Dictionary for GI and Hepatology (pp 216-217).
© 2014 Taylor & Francis Group.

Use this mnemonic:

AminoTransferases Increase Acutely By Many Causes Before Fulminant Disease Starts

- A = Autoimmune
- T = Tylenol (Acetaminophen)
- I = Ischemia
- A= Hepatitis A
- B = Hepatitis B (with or without hepatitis D superinfection or less likely coinfection)
- M = Mushroom *(Amanita phylloides)*
- C = Cocaine
- B = Budd-Chiari syndrome
- F = Fatty liver of pregnancy
- D = Drug-induced liver injury (eg, antibiotics, nonsteroidal anti-inflammatory drugs, anticonvulsants)
- S = Supplements (eg, black cohosh, kava kava, ephedra, pennyroyal)

Cutaneous Manifestations of Liver Disease

Anatomical Location	Examination Finding	Clinical Considerations
Face/head	Facial lipodystrophy	Alcohol
	Rhinophyma	Alcohol
	Rosacea	Alcohol
	Scleral icterus	Elevated bilirubin
	Lichen planopilaris	Hepatitis C
	Xanthelasmas	Primary biliary cirrhosis
Chest	Gynecomastia	Cirrhosis
	Spider angiomas	Portal hypertension
Abdomen	Striae	Ascites
	Caput medusae/ dilated abdominal wall veins	Portal hypertension
Upper extremity	Dupuytren's contracture	Alcohol
	Palmar erythema	Cirrhosis
	Terry's nails	Cirrhosis
	Clubbing	Cirrhosis

Fenkel JM, ed.
Quick Reference Dictionary for GI and Hepatology (pp 218-219).
© 2014 Taylor & Francis Group.

Anatomical Location	Examination Finding	Clinical Considerations
Upper extremity	Leukonychia	Cirrhosis
	Loss of axillary hair	Cirrhosis
	Muerhrcke's nails	Hypoalbuminemia
Lower extremity	Edema	Cirrhosis/portal hypertension
	Leukocytoclastic vasculitis	Cryoglobulinemia, vasculitis
Any location	Disseminated superficial porokeratosis	Alcohol
	Bier spots	Cirrhosis
	Jaundice	Cirrhosis
	Ecchymosis	Coagulopathy
	Lichen planus	Hepatitis C
	Prurigo nodularis	Hepatitis C
	Vitilgo	Hepatitis C while taking interferon treatment
	Bronze discoloration	Hemochromatosis
	Hyperpigmentation	Hemochromatosis
	Ichthyosiform alterations	Hemochromatosis

Selection Criteria for Liver Transplantation in Patients With Hepatocellular Carcinoma

In patients with hepatocellular carcinoma (HCC) and cirrhosis, liver transplantation offers the best chance for a cure because it removes both the tumor and the cirrhotic tissue from which new tumors can form. When transplantation was initially performed for HCC, 5-year survival rates were 30% to 40%. It was then determined that the tumor stage at the time of transplant influenced survival rates. The first tumor scoring system used was the Tumor Node Metastasis staging.

THE MILAN CRITERIA

Today, the most widely used criteria is the Milan Criteria. In 2002, the United Network of Organ Sharing deemed the Milan Criteria as the optimal criteria to determine appropriate use of liver transplantation in patients with HCC. Patients whose tumors fall within the criteria are deemed appropriate candidates for liver transplantation. Criteria include the following:

- A single HCC tumor smaller than 5 cm in greatest dimension

- Three or fewer tumors, with no single tumor larger than 3 cm in greatest dimension

- Absence of vascular invasion

Fenkel JM, ed.
Quick Reference Dictionary for GI and Hepatology (pp 220-221).
© 2014 Taylor & Francis Group.

THE UNIVERSITY OF CALIFORNIA, SAN FRANCISCO CRITERIA

Another set of criteria is described by physicians at the University of California, San Francisco, in which a more liberal set of criteria for transplantation was established. When initially described, those patients transplanted within the criteria had a 1-year survival rate of 90% and a 5-year survival rate of 75.2%. Criteria include the following:

- A single HCC 6.5 cm or smaller

- Three or fewer tumors, with the largest 4.5 cm or smaller, and a total tumor burden of 8 cm or smaller in diameter

- Absence of vascular invasion

For patients who have a tumor burden beyond the above criteria, locoregional therapies can be used to decrease the viable tumor burden so that it is within criteria (termed *down-staging*) to potentially allow for liver transplantation.

BIBLIOGRAPHY

Mazzaferro V, Regalia E, Doci R, et al. Liver transplantation for the treatment of small hepatocellular carcinomas in patients with cirrhosis. *N Engl J Med.* 1996;334:693-699.

Yao FY. Liver transplantation for hepatocellular carcinoma: beyond the Milan criteria. *Am J Transpl.* 2008;8:1982-1998.

Yao FY, Ferrell L, Bass NM, et al. Liver transplantation for HCC: expansion of the tumor size limits does not adversely impact survival. *Hepatology.* 2001;33:1394-1403.

Hepatitis C Virus Treatment Protocol

The treatment of chronic hepatitis C virus (HCV) is undergoing a major paradigm shift from interferon-based treatment regimens to interferon-free treatment regimens. Between 2011 and 2014, four new direct-acting antiviral (DAA) medications were approved by the Federal Drug Administration (FDA). At the time of publication, 15 to 20 new DAA medications are expected to compete for FDA approval in the next 4 to 5 years. Recommended treatment protocols are expected to change frequently as new medications come to market. Rapid guidelines jointly developed by the American Association for the Study of Liver Diseases (AASLD) and the Infectious Diseases Society of America (IDSA) are available at www.hcvguidelines.org. They are expected to be updated soon after each new medication approval, or as new data becomes available. Telaprevir and boceprevir are no longer recommended for use in any patients after the approval of sofosbuvir and simeprevir in December 2013, but historical treatment algorithms for HCV treatment naïve patients are included in this appendix for comparison to the newest treatments.

Fenkel JM, ed.
Quick Reference Dictionary for GI and Hepatology (pp 222-225).
© 2014 Taylor & Francis Group.

HCV GENOTYPE 1
TREATMENT PROTOCOL

P, Pegylated interferon; R, Ribavirin; SOF, Sofosbuvir; SIM, Simeprevir; T, Telaprevir; B, Boceprevir; (Number), Weeks; SVR, sustained virologic response

NAÏVE TO TREATMENT – INTERFERON-ELIGIBLE		
Options	**Duration, Weeks**	**Predicted SVR, %**
1. Triple Therapy P/R/SOF	12	90
2. Triple Therapy P/R/SIM (12) + P/R (12)	24	80
3. Triple Therapy P/R/T* – Response-guided: P/R/T (12) + P/R (12) P/R/T (12) + P/R (36)	24- 48	80
4. Triple Therapy P/R/B* – Response-guided: P/R (4) + P/R/B (24) P/R (4) + P/R/B (32) + P/R(12)	28-48	65
3. P/R (48)*	48	30-50
* Not recommended by current guidelines		

NAÏVE TO TREATMENT – INTERFERON-INELIGIBLE		
(as defined by www.hcvguidelines.org: prior intolerance to P, autoimmune hepatitis or other autoimmune disease, decompensated liver disease, history of major depression or clinical features consistent with depression, baseline neutropenia (neutrophils < 1500/uL), thrombocytopenia (platelets < 90,000/uL), anemia (hemoglobin < 10/uL), history of preexisting cardiac disease)		
Options	**Duration, Weeks**	**Predicted SVR, %**
1. SOF/SIM ± R #	12	> 90
2. SOF/R	24	60-70
# Off-label usage of two approved medications (not FDA-approved in combination)		

RELAPSER TO PRIOR TREATMENT WITH P/R – TREAT AS IF PATIENT IS NAÏVE TO TREATMENT		
Options	Duration, Weeks	Predicted SVR, %
1. Triple Therapy P/R/SOF	12	90
2. Triple Therapy P/R/SIM (12) + P/R (12)	24	80

PARTIAL NON-RESPONDERS TO P/R (2 LOG DROP AT WEEK 12, BUT NEVER ACHIEVED COMPLETE VIRAL SUPPRESSION) OR NULL RESPONDERS TO P/R (< 2 LOG DROP AT WEEK 12 OF TREATMENT)		
Options	Duration, Weeks	Predicted SVR, %
1. SOF/SIM ± R #	12	> 90
2. P/R/SOF	12	70
3. P/R/SIM (12) + P/R (12)	24	50-60
# Off-label usage of two approved medications (not FDA-approved in combination)		

HCV GENOTYPE 2
TREATMENT PROTOCOL

P, Pegylated interferon; R, Ribavirin; SOF, Sofosbuvir

NAÏVE TO TREATMENT OR PRIOR TREATMENT FAILURE		
Options	Duration, Weeks	Predicted SVR, %
1. R/SOF	12	> 90
2. P/R*	24	70-80
* Not recommended by current guidelines		

HCV GENOTYPE 3
TREATMENT PROTOCOL

P, Pegylated interferon; R, Ribavirin; SOF, Sofosbuvir

NAÏVE TO TREATMENT OR PRIOR TREATMENT FAILURE		
Options	**Duration, Weeks**	**Predicted SVR, %**
1. R/SOF	24	80
2. P/R/SOF	12	80
3. P/R*	24	60-70
* Not recommended by current guidelines		

HCV GENOTYPE 4
TREATMENT PROTOCOL

P, Pegylated interferon; R, Ribavirin; SOF, Sofosbuvir; SIM, Simeprevir; (Number), Weeks

NAÏVE TO TREATMENT OR PRIOR TREATMENT FAILURE		
Options	**Duration, Weeks**	**Predicted SVR, %**
1. P/R/SOF	12	>90
2. R/SOF	24	>80
3. P/R/SIM (12) + P/R (12)	24	>65
4. PR (48)*	48	60
* Not recommended by current guidelines		

Scoring Systems for Alcoholic Hepatitis

Alcoholic hepatitis is a severe form of liver disease seen in approximately 30% of heavy drinkers and can have mortality rates of 30% to 50%. Several scoring systems currently exist to identify patients with more severe disease and a higher risk of death.

DISCRIMINANT FUNCTION (DF) (ALSO CALLED MADDREY'S DISCRIMINANT FUNCTION)

- First scoring system developed.

- Described in a placebo-controlled trial to assess the benefit of corticosteroid use in patients with alcoholic hepatitis.

- The most widely used prognostic tool for mortality in patients with alcoholic hepatitis.

- After initial description in 1978, a modification was made in 1989.

  ○ The modified DF equation:
    DF = {4.6 * (patient's prothrombin time [PT] – control PT)} + total bilirubin

DF score greater than 32 indicates severe alcoholic hepatitis and has a 50% mortality rate; this is the threshold at which corticosteroid treatment should be initiated.

Jonathan M. Fenkel
Quick Reference Dictionary for GI and Hepatology (pp 226-229).
© 2014 Taylor & Francis Group.

MODEL FOR END-STAGE LIVER DISEASE (MELD) SCORE

MELD has been applied to patients with alcoholic hepatitis because the DF was believed to be a poor indicator of adverse events when applied clinically.

- The MELD score was developed initially to assess mortality for transjugular intrahepatic portosystemic shunt.

- It is the current system used to rank patients on the liver transplant list.

- The MELD score is calculated using the following formula: MELD = 3.78(Log^n serum bilirubin [mg/dL]) + 11.2(Log^n international normalized ratio [INR]) + 9.57(Log^n serum creatinine [mg/dL]) + 6.43

- Found to be a good predictor of mortality in patients with alcoholic hepatitis, but no values were deemed useful to stratify patients as being of low, intermediate, or high risk for poor outcomes.

- Not proven as useful in risk stratification.

GLASGOW ALCOHOLIC HEPATITIS SCORE (GAHS)

Developed in 2005 to better assess outcomes in patients with alcoholic hepatitis.

	Score		
Variable	**1**	**2**	**3**
Age (years)	< 50	≥ 50	
White blood cell count (109/L)	< 15	≥ 15	
Urea (mmol/L)	< 5	≥ 5	
INR	< 1.5	1.5 to 2.0	> 2.0
Bilirubin (μmol/L)	< 125	125 to 250	> 250

Score measured on day 1:

- ○ A score <9 predicts a 87% survival at 28 days and a 79% survival at day 84.

- ○ A score ≥9 predicts a 46% survival at 28 days and a 40% survival at day 84.

- Score measured between days 6 and 9:

  - ○ A score <9 predicts a 93% survival at 28 days and an 86% survival at day 84.

  - ○ A score ≥9 predicts a 47% survival at 28 days and a 37% survival at day 84.

LILLE MODEL

First developed in 2007 to predict 6-month survival in patients with alcoholic hepatitis who were taking corticosteroid treatment. Patients were checked on day 7 of corticosteroid treatment.

- Lille Model = 3.19 − 0.101 * (age [years]) + 0.147 * (day 0 albumin [g/L]) + 0.0165 * (change in bilirubin from day 0 to 7 [µM]) − 0.206 * (renal insufficiency) − 0.0065 * (day 0 total bilirubin [µM]) − 0.0096 * (prothrombin time [seconds]).\

  - ○ Renal insufficiency rated as 0 if absent and 1 if present.

  - ○ A score >0.45 predicts a 6-month mortality of 25%±3.8%.

  - ○ A score <0.45 predicts a 6-month mortality of 85%±2.5%.

  - ○ Therefore, patients with a score >0.45 were unlikely to benefit from continued corticosteroid therapy and deemed nonresponders; their participation should be stopped.

ABIC (AGE, SERUM BILIRUBIN, INR AND SERUM CREATININE) SCORE

Described in 2008 as a tool to predict the short- and long-term mortality of patients with alcoholic hepatitis. It is calculated within the first 48 hours of admission.

- ABIC = (age * 0.1) + (serum bilirubin * 0.08) + (serum creatinine * 0.3) + (INR * 0.8)

- Patients are stratified into low, intermediate, and high risk categories.

    ○ ABIC score < 6.71 had a 100% survival rate at 90 days and a 97.1% survival rate at 1 year in original study.

    ○ Follow-up studies suggest mortality up to 20% with score < 6.71.

    ○ ABIC score ≥ 9 had a 33.3% one-year survival.

BIBLIOGRAPHY

Dominguez M, Rincón D, Abraldes JG, et al. A new scoring system for prognostic stratification of patients with alcoholic hepatitis. *Am J Gastroenterol.* 2008;103:2747-2756.

Dunn W, Jamil LH, Brown LS, et al. MELD accurately predicts mortality in patients with alcoholic hepatitis. *Hepatology.* 2005;41:353-358.

Forrest EH, Evans CD, Stewart S, et al. Analysis of factors predictive of mortality in alcoholic hepatitis and derivation and validation of the Glasgow alcoholic hepatitis score. *Gut.* 2005;54;1174-1179.

Forrest EH, Fisher NC, Singhal S, et al. Comparison of the Glasgow alcoholic hepatitis score and the ABIC score for the assessment of alcoholic hepatitis. *Am J Gastroenterol.* 2010;105:701-702.

Forrest EH, Morris AJ, Stewart S, et al. The Glasgow alcoholic hepatitis score identifies patients who may benefit from corticosteroids. *Gut.* 2007;56:1743-1746.

Louvet, A, Naveau, S, Abdelnour, M, et al. The Lille model: a new tool for therapeutic strategy in patients with severe alcoholic hepatitis treated with steroids. *Hepatology.* 2007;45:1348-1354.

Lucey MR, Mathurin P, Morgan TR. Alcoholic hepatitis. *N Engl J Med.* 2009;360:2758-2769.

Maddrey WC, Boitnott JK, Bedine MS, Weber FL Jr, Mezey E, White RI Jr. Corticosteroid therapy of alcoholic hepatitis. *Gastroenterology.* 1978;75:193-199.

Scoring System for Autoimmune Hepatitis

Autoimmune hepatitis affects a variety of patients, and its clinical presentation can be heterogeneous. Due to its high mortality rate and no single accurate diagnostic test, the International Autoimmune Hepatitis Group devised diagnostic criteria in 1993, which were then revised in 1999.

DIAGNOSTIC SCORING SYSTEM FOR AUTOIMMUNE HEPATITIS IN ADULTS

Variable	Score
Gender	
Female	+2
Alk Phos: AST (or ALT) ratio	
>3	−2
<1.5	+2
γ-globulin or IgG level (times above the upper limit of normal)	
>2.0	+3
1.5 to 2.0	+2
1.0 to 1.5	+1
<1.0	0

Fenkel JM, ed.
Quick Reference Dictionary for GI and Hepatology (pp 230-233).
© 2014 Taylor & Francis Group.

Variable	Score
Antibody titers (ANA, ASM, or anti-LKM1)	
> 1:80	+3
1:80	+2
1:40	+1
< 1:40	0
AMA positive	−4
Other auto-antibodies associated with liver disease	+2
Markers of active viral hepatitis infection	
Positive	−3
Negative	+3
Use of hepatotoxic drugs	
Yes	−4
No	+1
Alcohol consumption	
< 25 gm/day	+2
> 60 gm/day	−2
Concurrent nonhepatic autoimmune disease	
Yes	+2
Histologic features	
Inferface hepatitis	+3
Plasma cell infiltrate	1
Rosettes	+1
None of the above	−5
Biliary changes	−3
Atypical features	−3
HLA	
DR3 or DR4	+1

Variable	Score
Response to corticosteroid treatment	
Remission	+2
Remission with relapse	+3

Alk Phos, alkaline phosphatase; AST, aspartate aminotransferase; ALT, alanine aminotransferase; ASM, anti-smooth muscle antibody; anti-LKM1, anti-liver kidney microsomal antibody 1; HLA, human leukocyte antigen.

A diagnosis of autoimmune hepatitis is made if the patients' score is higher than 15 prior to corticosteroid treatment or higher than 17 after corticosteroid administration. Sensitivity ranges from 97% to 100%, and specificity (when patients with chronic hepatitis C are excluded) ranges from 66% to 92%. In cholestatic syndromes with autoimmune features, the sensitivity ranges from 45% to 65%.

Due to the complex nature of the above criteria, a simplified diagnostic criteria for routine clinical practice was devised by the International Autoimmune Hepatitis Group in 2008.

SIMPLIFIED DIAGNOSTIC CRITERIA

Variable	Score
Autoantibodies	
ANA or ASM ≥ 1:40	1
ANA or ASM ≥ 1:80	1
Or anti-LKM1 ≥ 1:40	2
Or SLA/LP positive	2
IgG level	
More than the upper limit of normal	1
> 1.10 times the upper limit of normal	2

Variable	Score
Liver histology	
Compatible with AIH	1
Typical AIH	2
Absence of viral hepatitis	2

ANA, antinuclear antibody; ASM, anti-smooth muscle antibody; LKM1, anti-liver kidney microsomal antibody 1; SLA/LP, soluble liver/liver-pancreas antibody; AIH, autoimmune hepatitis.

A score of 6 or more indicates a probable diagnosis of autoimmune hepatitis (88% sensitive and 97% specific) and a score of 7 or more indicates a definitive diagnosis of autoimmune hepatitis (81% sensitive and 99% specific).

BIBLIOGRAPHY

Alvarez F, Berg PA, Bianchi FB, et al. International Autoimmune Hepatitis Group report: review of criteria for diagnosis of autoimmune hepatitis. *J Hepatol.* 1999;31:929-938.

Hennes EM, Zeniya M, Czaja AJ, et al. Simplified criteria for the diagnosis of autoimmune hepatitis. *Hepatology.* 2008;48:169-176.

Johnson PJ, McFarlane IG. Meeting Report: International Autoimmune Hepatitis Group. *Hepatology.* 1993;18:998-1005.

Targets of Transplant Immunosuppression

IMMUNOLOGY PRIMER

The primary goal of liver transplant immunosuppression is to prevent acute and chronic graft rejection that cause graft loss. Rejection is a host T-cell–mediated process. Foreign antigens in the graft are circulated to secondary lymphoid organs after reperfusion. Antigen presenting cells (APCs) process antigens and sensitize naïve T-cells via major histocompatibility complex–T-cell receptor (TCR) interaction. This interaction induces the cascade of T-cell activation, clonal expansion, and graft inflammation. To a lesser extent, circulating T-cells may be exposed to a foreign antigen within the graft, with Kupffer cells acting as APCs.

T-cells require 3 signals for maturation. Knowing these 3 signals, we can better understand the potential targets for immunosuppressive therapy. Seven potential targets exist currently.

- Signal 1: The APC presents an antigen to the TCR.

  - Target 1: Block TCR engagement with APC

    - Medications: anti-thymocyte globulin, muronomab

- Signal 2: Costimulation between ligands on the APC and T-cell is required to initiate calcineurin to begin the process of upregulating production of interleukin-2 (IL-2) and

Fenkel JM, ed.
Quick Reference Dictionary for GI and Hepatology (pp 234-235).
© 2014 Taylor & Francis Group.

other cytokines. IL-2 is the most important cytokine in this cascade.

- ○ Target 2: Block costimulation of APC/T-cell engagement
  - ᴧ Medication: belatacept
- ○ Target 3: Block calcineurin pathway
  - ᴧ Medications: tacrolimus, cyclosporine
- ○ Target 4: Inhibit IL-2 production
  - ᴧ Medication: glucocorticoids
- Signal 3: IL-2 then acts in an autocrine fashion to stimulate the T-cell to begin proliferation and synthesis of other cytokines via mammalian target or rapamycin (mTOR) pathway.
  - ○ Target 5: Block IL-2 from reentering the cell via IL-2R
    - ᴧ Medication: basiliximab
  - ○ Target 6: Block mTOR pathway
    - ᴧ Medications: sirolimus, everolimus
  - ○ Target 7: Block nucleotide synthesis
    - ᴧ Medications: mycophenolate mofetil, mycophenolic acid, azathioprine

Elevated Liver Function Tests in Pregnancy

Figure 8-1. Abnormal liver tests in pregnancy.

Determine if abnormal liver tests are physiologic changes of pregnancy

Liver-related tests that are affected by pregnancy:
Increased: Alkaline phosphatase, WBC count, alpha-fetoprotein
Unchanged: AST, ALT, PT, bilirubin, platelets
Decreased: Albumin, hemoglobin

If unexplained by physiologic changes consider relationship to pregnancy

Pregnancy-related liver diseases
Hyperemesis gravidarum (HG)
Intrahepatic cholestasis of pregnancy (ICP)
Pre-eclampsia and eclampsia
HELLP syndrome
Acute fatty liver of pregnancy (AFLP)

Pregnancy-unrelated liver diseases
Pre-existing liver disease
Cirrhosis and portal hypertension
Chronic Hepatitis B and C
Autoimmune liver disease
Wilson's disease
PBC
PSC
Non-alcoholic fatty liver disease

Liver disease co-incident with pregnancy
Viral hepatitis (A, B/D, C, E)
Drug-induced hepatotoxicity
Gallstones
Budd-Chiari syndrome
Liver transplantation

Fenkel JM, ed.
Quick Reference Dictionary for GI and Hepatology (pp 236-238).
© 2014 Taylor & Francis Group.

Pregnancy-related liver diseases

	Trimester	Presentation	Laboratory Data	Histology
HG	1,2	N/V, wt loss, nutritional deficiency	↑ Bilirubin (×4 ULN), ↑ ALT/AST (×2–4 ULN)	No distinct pathology
ICP	1,2,3	Pruritis, jaundice, A/P	↑ Bilirubin (×6 ULN), ↑ ALT/AST (×6 ULN), ↑ serum bile acids	Centrilobular cholestasis
Pre-eclampsia	2,3	HTN, edema, proteinuria, neurologic sxs	↑ Bilirubin (×2–5 ULN), ↑ ALT/AST (×10–50 ULN), ↓ platelets	Periportal hemorrhage, Necrosis, fibrin deposits
HELLP	2,3	A/P, N/V, edema, HTN, proteinuria	↑ ALT/AST (×10–20 ULN), ↑ LDH, ↓ platelets, ↑ uric acid, hemolytic anemia	Periportal hemorrhage, Necrosis, fibrin deposits
AFLP	2,3	A/P, N/V, fatigue, jaundice	↑ Bilirubin (×6 × 8 ULN), ↑ ALT/AST (×5–10 ULN), hypoglycemia often	Microvesicular fat

Figure 8-2. Pregnancy related liver diseases. N/V, nausea/vomiting; ULN, upper limit of normal; A/P, abdominal pain; HTN, hypertension; sxs, symptoms; LDH, lactate dehydrogenase.

BIBLIOGRAPHY

Joshi D, James A, Quaglia A, Westbrook RH, Heneghan MA. Liver disease in pregnancy. *Lancet.* 2010;375:594-605.

Pan C, Perumalswami PV. Pregnancy-related liver diseases. *Clin Liver Dis.* 2011;15:199-208.

Triggers for
Hepatic Encephalopathy

Hepatic encephalopathy (HE) is a neuropsychiatric disorder seen with acute or chronic liver failure. In most cases, a precipitating event can be identified through a detailed history and evaluation; however, in up to 20% of cases, an etiology may not be identified. Common causes of HE are listed below.

1. Infection

   a. Spontaneous bacterial peritonitis

   b. Urinary tract infection

   c. Pneumonia

   d. Cellulitis

2. Bacteremia

   a. Dietary indiscretion

   b. Increased sodium intake

   c. Increased protein intake

   d. Increased free water intake leading to hyponatremia

   e. Alcohol use

3. Hepatic insult/injury

   a. Increased portosystemic venous shunting

      i. Transjugular intrahepatic portosystemic shunt placement

Fenkel JM, ed.
Quick Reference Dictionary for GI and Hepatology (pp 239-241).
© 2014 Taylor & Francis Group.

      ii. Portal vein thrombosis

  b. Surgery

  c. Acute or chronic injury

      i. Drug-induced

      ii. Acute viral hepatitis

      iii. Toxin-induced (eg, cocaine, alcohol)

  d. New hepatocellular carcinoma

4. Medication

  a. Noncompliance with HE medications (eg, rifaximin, lactulose)

  b. Central nervous system medications (eg, anesthesia, sedatives)

      i. Benzodiazepines

      ii. Narcotics/analgesics

  c. Overuse of diuretics, lactulose, or other laxatives causing dehydration

5. Increased nitrogenous load

  a. Gastrointestinal bleeding

  b. Severe constipation

  c. Excessive dietary protein

6. Metabolic disturbance

  a. Hypokalemia

  b. Renal insufficiency

      i. Hepatorenal syndrome

      ii. Acute tubular necrosis

      iii. Urinary tract infection

      iv. Allergic interstitial nephritis

  c. Alkalosis

d. Hyponatremia

e. Hypomagnesemia

f. Dehydration

   i. Excessive diuresis

   ii. Diarrhea

   iii. Vomiting

   iv. Inadequate oral hydration

g. Hypoxia

   i. Sleep apnea

   ii. Pneumonia

   iii. Pleural effusion (hepatic hydrothorax)

   iv. Hepatopulmonary syndrome

BIBLIOGRAPHY

Butterworth RF. Complications of cirrhosis III. Hepatic encephalopathy. *J Hepatol.* 2000;32:171-180.

Ferenci P, Lockwood A, Mullen K, Tarter R, Weissenborn K, Blei AT. Hepatic encephalopathy—definition, nomenclature, diagnosis, and quantification: final report of the working party at the 11th World Congresses of Gastroenterology, Vienna, 1998. *Hepatology.* 2002;35:716-721.

Häussinger D, Kircheis G, Fischer R, Schliess F, vom Dahl S. Hepatic encephalopathy in chronic liver disease: a clinical manifestation of astrocyte swelling and low-grade cerebral edema? *J Hepatol.* 2000;32:6:1035-1038.

Munoz SJ. Hepatic encephalopathy. *Med Clin North Am.* 2008;92:795-812.

Approach to Elevated Liver Enzyme Tests

Abnormal liver enzyme tests are common in clinical practice. More than 20% of ambulatory medical patients have an elevated alanine aminotransferase (ALT) level, and more than 3% have an abnormal alkaline phosphatase (AlkPh) level. It is important to determine the etiology of the elevated tests because chronic liver disease may be present, and identification with correctable action can prevent cirrhosis or liver failure in the future. Following these 5 steps can help make the most accurate diagnosis.

Step 1: Confirm the Test Result. Liver enzyme tests can be affected by hemolysis of a blood specimen, so confirmation should always be the first step taken.

Step 2: History and Physical Examination. Many causes of elevated liver enzymes can be elicited through a detailed history and examination.

- Medication and over-the-counter/herbal supplements: Of particular interest are antiepileptics, cholesterol-lowering medications, antibiotics, antituberculosis drugs, oral contraceptives, chronic use of acetaminophen or products containing ibuprofen, and herbal supplements, such as kava kava, black cohosh, and pennyroyal.

- Past medical/surgical history: Identify comorbidities that may predispose patients to liver injury or require medications that might. In particular, does the patient have risk

Fenkel JM, ed.
Quick Reference Dictionary for GI and Hepatology (pp 242-245).
© 2014 Taylor & Francis Group.

factors for nonalcoholic fatty liver disease, including diabetes mellitus, hypertension, coronary artery disease, obesity, or hyperlipidemia; recent hospitalizations; or recent parenteral nutrition?

- Social history: Quantify alcohol use on a daily, weekly, monthly, and lifetime basis; evaluate for risk factors for viral hepatitis (ie, illicit drug use, tattoos, needle sharing, transfusions, multiple sexual partners).

- Family history: Identify risk for hereditary conditions, including hemochromatosis, alpha-1 antitrypsin deficiency, Wilson's disease, and polycystic liver disease.

- Occupational history: Toxic exposures, military experience, needlesticks.

- Travel history: Ingestion of Jamaican bush tea, African iron overload, and Lyme disease.

- Examination evidence of chronic liver disease: Spider angiomas, caput medusae, palmar erythema, Dupuytren's contractures, ascites, hepatosplenomegaly, asterixis, and jaundice.

- Extrahepatic manifestations of liver disease: Rashes (eg, leukocytoclastic vasculitis, lichen planus), psychiatric disease (Wilson's disease), renal failure (hepatitis B/C), Sjogren's syndrome (primary biliary cirrhosis).

Step 3: Data Collection and Categorization. The laboratory tests and imaging studies ordered should be tailored to the most likely diagnoses as determined from Step 2. Categorizing is also helpful in deciding which studies to order. Try categorizing into these options:

- Hepatocellular versus cholestatic (hepatocellular usually increased aspartate aminotransferase (AST)/ALT >> AlkPh whereas cholestatic usually increased AlkPh >> AST/ALT).

  ○ Acute versus chronic hepatocellular

  ○ Intrahepatic versus extrahepatic cholestatic

- Symptomatic versus asymptomatic

- Isolated hyperbilirubinemia (increased total bilirubin, others normal)

- Common laboratory tests ordered include the following: complete blood count (CBC), comprehensive metabolic panel (CMP), direct bilirubin, prothrombin time/international normalized ratio, viral hepatitis panel (Hep A total Ab, HepBsAg, HepBsab, HepBcAb [total], Hep Cab), anti-nuclear antibody (ANA), anti-mitochondrial antibody (AMA), anti-smooth muscle Ab (ASMA), iron studies (iron, total iron binding capacity, ferritin, iron saturation), ceruloplasmin level, hemoglobin A1C (if diabetes mellitus is suspected or known), celiac disease panel, and thyroid stimulating hormone.

- Obtain a right upper quadrant ultrasound to look for biliary disease, to assess for presence or absence of cirrhosis or liver masses, and to evaluate grossly for fatty liver disease.

- Evaluate the data:

  ○ Abnormal celiac disease panel: Should prompt further workup with upper endoscopy for biopsies to evaluate for celiac disease.

  ○ Elevated ANA: Titers greater than 1:160 should prompt further work-up for primary biliary cirrhosis, autoimmune hepatitis, and primary sclerosing cholangitis.

  ○ Elevated AMA: Raises concern for primary biliary cirrhosis.

  ○ Elevated iron studies: Raises concern for hemochromatosis.

  ○ Low ceruloplasmin: Raises concern for Wilson's disease.

  ○ Elevated ASMA: Titers greater than 1:160 raise suspicion for autoimmune hepatitis.

  ○ Viral hepatitis serologies: Can lead to inclusion or exclusion of hepatitis A/B/C/D as possible etiologies of elevated liver enzyme tests.

- ○ Fatty liver on ultrasound: Could indicate nonalcoholic steatohepatitis or alcohol-related hepatitis or, rarely, be seen in viral hepatitis C.

- ○ Obstruction on ultrasound: Proceed with endoscopic retrograde cholangiopancreatography or magnetic resonance cholangiopancreatography.

- Cross-sectional imaging if ultrasound results are equivocal or negative and diagnosis still unexplained.

- Liver biopsy if above workup is negative.

Step 4: Specific Diagnosis. Steps 2 and 3 should lead to a specific diagnosis. If no cause is obvious, repeat Step 2 and consider testing for more rare causes of elevated liver tests, repeating a liver biopsy, or having the slides interpreted by another pathologist. If alcohol use is clouding the specific diagnosis, alcohol should be withheld for at least 1 month and then the tests should be repeated and the diagnosis reassessed.

Step 5: Implement Therapy. Treatment is directed at the cause of the elevated liver tests. If toxins, herbals, or medications are suspected, then a therapeutic trial off medications can be done. The liver enzymes can then be rechecked in a few weeks and reassessed for resolution. If fatty liver disease is suspected, then weight loss and optimization of underlying risk factors is paramount. Antiviral therapy exists for hepatitis B and C. Alcohol cessation again should be incorporated into all treatment plans because it can cloud therapeutic response and diagnosis.

Interpretation of Hepatitis B Serological Markers

Diagnosis	HBsAg	HBsAb	HBcAb (total)	HBc IgM	HBeAg	HBeAb	HBV DNA (IU/mL)	ALT
Acute HBV	+	–	+	+	+	±	High	High
Resolved HBV (natural HBV immunity)	–	+	+	–	–	±	Absent	Normal
HBV immune by vaccination	–	+	–	–	–	–	Absent	Normal
HBV reactivation	+	–	+	±	+	±	>20,000	High
Chronic: HBeAg positive								
Immune tolerance phase	+	–	+	–	+	–	>20,000	Normal

Fenkel JM, ed.
Quick Reference Dictionary for GI and Hepatology (pp 246–247).
© 2014 Taylor & Francis Group.

Diagnosis	HBsAg	HBsAb	HBcAb (total)	HBc IgM	HBeAg	HBeAb	HBV DNA (IU/mL)	ALT
Immune active (clearance) phase	+	-	+	-	+	±	>20,000	High
Chronic: HBeAg negative								
Immune control phase (inactive carrier)	+	-	+	-	-	+	<2,000	Normal
Immune escape phase (often associated with mutated virus)	+	-	+	-	-	+	>2,000	High

HBsAg, Hepatitis B surface antigen; HBsAb, Hepatitis B surface antibody; HBcAb, Hepatitis B core antibody total; HBc IgM, Hepatitis B core IgM (Immunoglobulin M) antibody; HBeAg, Hepatitis B e-antigen; HBeAb, Hepatitis B e-antibody; HBV DNA, Hepatitis B virus DNA (deoxyribonucleic acid); IU, international units; ALT, alanine aminotransferase.

GI/Luminal

Grading of Erosive Esophagitis

The two most frequently used grading systems to assess the severity and healing of erosive esophagitis are the Los Angeles classification and the Savary-Miller classification.

Los Angeles (LA) Classification

- LA Class A: One or more mucosal breaks each no longer than 5 mm.

- LA Class B: At least one mucosal break more than 5 mm in length but not continuous between the tops of adjacent mucosal folds.

- LA Class C: At least one continuous mucosal break between tops of adjacent mucosal folds but not circumferential.

- LA Class D: Circumferential mucosal break.

Savary-Miller Classification

- Grade I: One or more non-confluent reddish spots, with or without exudates.

- Grade II: Erosive and exudative lesions in the distal esophagus that can be confluent but not circumferential.

- Grade III: Circumferential erosions in distal esophagus covered by hemorrhage and pseudomembranous exudates.

- Grade IV: Presence of complications, including deep ulcers, scarring with Barrett's metaplasia, or stenosis/stricture.

Fenkel JM, ed.
Quick Reference Dictionary for GI and Hepatology (pp 249-250).
© 2014 Taylor & Francis Group.

BIBLIOGRAPHY

Armstrong D, Bennett JR, Blum A, et al. The endoscopic assessment of esophagitis: a progress report on observer agreement. *Gastroenterology*. 1996;111:85-92.

Dent J. Endoscopic grading of reflux oesophagitis: the past, present and future. *Best Pract Res Clin Gastroenterol*. 2008;22:585-599.

Yaghoobi M, Padol S, Yuan Y, Hunt RH. Impact of oesophagitis classification in evaluating healing of erosive oesophagitis after therapy with proton pump inhibitors: a pooled analysis. *Eur J Gastroenterol Hepatol*. 2010;22:583-590.

Approach to Dysphagia

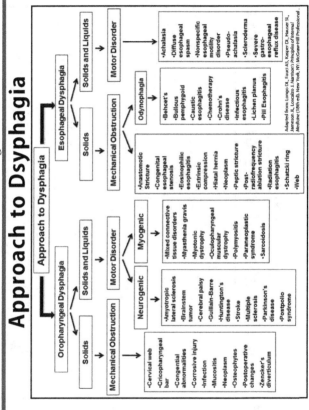

Approach to Dysphagia

Oropharyngeal Dysphagia

- Solids
  - **Mechanical Obstruction**
    - Cervical web
    - Cricopharyngeal bar
    - Congenital abnormalities
    - Corrosive injury
    - Infection
    - Mucositis
    - Neoplasm
    - Osteophytes
    - Postoperative changes
    - Zenker's diverticulum

- Solids and Liquids
  - **Motor Disorder**
    - **Neurogenic**
      - Amyotropic lateral sclerosis
      - Brainstem tumor
      - Cerebral palsy
      - Guillain-Barre
      - Huntington's disease
      - Stroke
      - Multiple sclerosis
      - Parkinson's disease
      - Postpolio syndrome
    - **Myogenic**
      - Mixed connective tissue disorders
      - Myasthenia gravis
      - Myotonic dystrophy
      - Oculopharyngeal muscular dystrophy
      - Polymyositis
      - Paraneoplastic syndrome
      - Sarcoidosis

Esophageal Dysphagia

- Solids
  - **Mechanical Obstruction**
    - Anastomotic Stricture
    - Congenital esophageal stenosis
    - Eosinophilic esophagitis
    - Extrinsic compression
    - Hiatal hernia
    - Neoplasm
    - Peptic stricture
    - Post-radiofrequency ablation stricture
    - Radiation esophagitis
    - Schatzki ring
    - Web
  - **Odynophagia**
    - Behcet's
    - Bullous pemphigoid
    - Caustic esophagitis
    - Chemotherapy
    - Crohn's disease
    - Infectious esophagitis
    - Lichen planus
    - Pill Esophagitis

- Solids and Liquids
  - **Motor Disorder**
    - Achalasia
    - Diffuse esophageal spasm
    - Nonspecific esophageal motility disorder
    - Pseudo-achalasia
    - Scleroderma
    - Severe gastro-esophageal reflux disease

Adapted from: Longo DL, Fauci AS, Kasper DL, Hauser SL, Jameson JL, Loscalzo J, Harrison's Principles of Internal Medicine (18th ed). New York, NY: McGraw-Hill Professional.

Fenkel JM, ed.
Quick Reference Dictionary for GI and Hepatology (pp 251).
© 2014 Taylor & Francis Group.

Thiopurine Methyltransferase Pathway

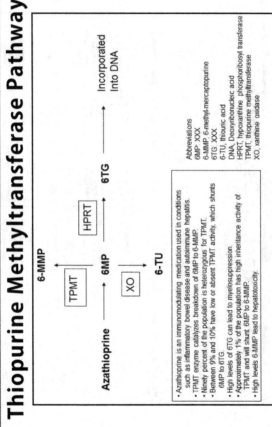

6-MMP

Azathioprine → 6MP → 6TG → Incorporated Into DNA

TPMT

HPRT

XO

6-TU

- Azathioprine is an immunomodulating medication used in conditions such as inflammatory bowel disease and autoimmune hepatitis.
- TPMT enzyme catalyzes breakdown of 6MP to 6-MMP.
- Ninety percent of the population is heterozygous for TPMT.
- Between 9% and 10% have low or absent TPMT activity, which shunts 6MP to 6TG.
- High levels of 6TG can lead to myelosuppression.
- Approximately 1% of the population has high inheritance activity of TPMT and will shunt 6MP to 6-MMP.
- High levels 6-MMP lead to hepatotoxicity.

Abbreviations
6MP: XXX
6-MMP: 6-methyl-mercaptopurine
6TG: XXX
6-TU: thiouric acid
DNA: Deoxyribonucleic acid
HPRT: hypoxanthine phosphoribosyl transferase
TPMT: thiopurine methyltransferase
XO: xanthine oxidase

Adapted from: Marsh S, Van Booven DJ. The increasing complexity of mercaptopurine pharmacogenomics. *Clin Pharmacol Ther.* 2009;85:139-141.

Jonathan M. Fenkel
Quick Reference Dictionary for GI and Hepatology (pp 252).
© 2014 Taylor & Francis Group.

Peptic Ulcer Disease Therapy and Rebleeding Rates

Peptic ulcer disease (PUD) is a common GI issue, and treatment is aimed at 3 areas: treating acute complications, healing the ulcer, and modifying underlying risk factors to prevent recurrence.

TREATING ACUTE COMPLICATIONS

The most life-threatening complications of PUD are intestinal perforation and gastrointestinal bleeding.

- Intestinal perforation

  ○ Presents as acute abdominal pain.

  ○ Surgical abdomen (diffuse severe tenderness, guarding, and rebound tenderness).

  ○ Radiographs or computed tomography scans will show free intraperitoneal air.

  ○ Surgical intervention is usually necessary.

- Gastrointestinal bleeding

  ○ Active, intermittent, or chronic gastrointestinal bleeding.

  ○ If PUD is suspected clinically, an intravenous proton pump inhibitor (PPI) bolus should be started and then followed by continues infusion.

Fenkel JM, ed.
Quick Reference Dictionary for GI and Hepatology (pp 253-256).
© 2014 Taylor & Francis Group.

- ○ Endoscopic examination is preferred over radiologic examination as the first-line examination because diagnosis and therapy can occur simultaneously.

- ○ Endoscopic hemostasis can be achieved with endoscopic electrocautery, clips, or the injection of epinephrine and is used in ulcers with a stigmata that predict a higher risk of rebleeding (eg, adherent clot, visible vessels, and active bleeding).

- ○ Risk of rebleeding with only medical therapy based on initial ulcer appearance:

  - ‣ Clean base = 5%

  - ‣ Flat spot = 10%

  - ‣ Adherent clot = 25%

  - ‣ Nonbleeding visible vessel = 50%

  - ‣ Active bleeding = 55% to 90%

- Rebleeding rates for high-risk lesions range from 5% to 20% with endoscopic therapy.

- Risk factors for rebleeding include the following:

  - ○ Size of the ulcer

  - ○ Location of the ulcer (lesser curvature is higher risk)

  - ○ Comorbid illnesses (particularly end-stage renal disease)

  - ○ Active bleeding at time of initial endoscopy

Healing the Ulcer

- Antisecretory therapy is the mainstay of medical management in the healing stage:

  - ○ PPI

  - ○ Histamine receptor antagonist (H2 blocker)

  - ○ Prefer oral (PPI) for 4 to 6 weeks

- Stop nonsteroidal anti-inflammatory drugs (NSAIDs) if implicated in etiology.

- Test for and treat *Helicobacter pylori* infection if present.
- Popular *H pylori* treatment regimens include the following:
  - PPI twice daily + clarithromycin 500 mg twice daily + amoxicillin 1000 mg twice daily for 10 to 14 days
  - PPI twice daily + clarithromycin 500 mg twice daily + metronidazole 500 mg twice daily for 10 to 14 days
  - PPI twice daily + bismuth subsalicylate 525 mg four times daily + metronidazole 250 mg four times daily + tetracycline 500 mg four times daily for 10 to 14 days
  - Levofloxacin 250 mg daily + omeprazole 40 mg daily + nitazoxanide 500 mg twice daily + doxycycline 100 mg nightly for 7 to 10 days; commonly known by the mnemonic LOAD
  - Levofloxacin 250 mg twice daily + amoxicillin 1000 mg twice daily + PPI twice daily for 14 days
- If the ulcer was in the stomach, most gastroenterologists will repeat an endoscopy in 2 to 3 months to document ulcer healing.
- Ulcers that are not completely healed after 8 weeks of appropriate treatment may represent malignancy, and biopsies should be performed.
- Consider workup for Zollinger-Ellison syndrome if ulcers remain unhealed after several months of adequate antisecretory therapy.

MODIFYING UNDERLYING RISK FACTORS TO PREVENT RECURRENCE

- *H pylori* eradication
- Avoidance of NSAIDs
- Alcohol cessation
- Tobacco cessation
- Avoid cocaine and methamphetamines

BIBLIOGRAPHY

Basu PP, Rayapudi K, PacanaT, Shah NJ, Krishnaswamy N, Flynn M. A randomized study comparing levofloxacin, omeprazole, nitazoxinide, and doxycline versus triple therapy for the eradication of Helicobacter pylori. *Am J Gastroenterol.* 2011;106:1970-1975.

Chey WD, Wong BC. American College of Gastroenterology guideline on the management of Helicobacter pylori infection. *Am J Gastroenterol.* 2007;102:1808-1825.

Gisbert JP, Calvet X. Review article: Helicobacter pylori-negative duodenal ulcer disease. *Aliment Pharmacol Ther.* 2009;30:791-815.

Gralnek IM, Barkun AN, Bardou M. Management of acute bleeding from a peptic ulcer. *N Engl J Med.* 2008;359:928-937.

Katschinski B, Logan R, Davies J, Faulkner G, Pearson J, Langman M. Prognostic factors in upper gastrointestinal bleeding. *Dig Dis Sci.* 1994;39:706-712.

Laine L, Peterson WL. Bleeding peptic ulcer. *N Engl J Med.* 1994;331:717-727.

Crohn's Disease Versus Ulcerative Colitis in Tabular Format

Distinguishing Features	Crohn's Disease (CD)	Ulcerative Colitis (UC)
Age of onset	Bimodal: 15 to 30 years or 60 to 80 years	Bimodal: 15 to 30 years or 60 to 80 years
At risk populations	Ashkenazi Jews, some genetic inheritance	Ashkenazi Jews, some genetic inheritance
Tobacco	Increases risk of disease	Decreases risk of disease
Location	Anywhere in GI tract but most often includes terminal ileum	Always involves the rectum but can involve the entire colon. Does not affect upper GI tract or small intestine
Anatomically continuous?	No; can have skip lesions	Yes

Fenkel, JM ed.
Quick Reference Dictionary for GI and Hepatology (pp 257-259).
© 2014 Taylor & Francis Group.

Distinguishing Features	Crohn's Disease (CD)	Ulcerative Colitis (UC)
Common clinical presentation	Fever, right lower quadrant pain, weight loss, diarrhea with or without blood	Hematochezia, tenesmus, abdominal pain, weight loss
Endoscopic findings	Deep ulcerations, aphthous ulceration, cobblestone appearance of intestines, noncontinuous involvement (skip lesions)	Superficial erosions and ulceration, continuous involvement of the GI tract; only involves colon
Biopsy findings	Transmural inflammation, cryptitis, granulomas	Inflammation limited to mucosa and submucosa, cryptitis, and crypt abscesses
Intestinal complications	Fistulas, strictures, bowel obstruction, perianal disease, cancer	Toxic megacolon, cancer
Extraintestinal manifestations	Erythema nodosum (CD>UC), pyoderma gangrenosum (UC>CD), primary sclerosing cholangitis (UC>CD), ankylosing spondylitis (CD>UC), sacroiliitis (CD=UC), uveitis, iritis, episcleritis	

Distinguishing Features	Crohn's Disease (CD)	Ulcerative Colitis (UC)
Risk for cancer?	Slightly increased	More increased
Treatment options	5-ASA compounds, steroids, antibiotics, azathioprine, 6-mercaptopurine, cyclosporine, biologics (eg, infliximab, adalimumab), total parenteral nutrition, surgery	5-ASA compounds, steroids, azathioprine, 6-mercaptopurine, cyclosporine, biologics (eg, infliximab, adalimumab), surgery
Curative with surgery?	No	Yes

Adapted from Friedman S, Blumberg RS. Inflammatory bowel disease. In: Longo DL, Fauci AS, Kasper DL, Hauser SL, Jameson JL, Loscalzo J, eds. *Harrison's Principles of Internal Medicine.* 18th ed. New York: McGraw-Hill Professional; 2012:2477-2495.

Differential Diagnosis of Terminal Ileitis

Not everything that affects the terminal ileum is Crohn's disease. Below is a table of other diseases to consider when evaluating the cause of terminal ileal inflammation.

Etiology	Differential Diagnosis
Inflammatory	Crohn's disease, backwash ileitis (from ulcerative colitis)
Infectious	*Actinomyces israelii, Clostridium difficile, Campylobacter* spp, *Cryptococcus neoformans, Cytomegalovirus, Histoplasma capsulatum,* human immunodeficiency virus, *Mycobacterium tuberculosis, Mycobacterium avium* complex, *Salmonella* spp, *Shigella* spp, *Yersinia enterocolitica, Yersinia pseudotuberculosis*
Infiltrative	Amyloidosis, endometriosis, eosinophilic gastroenteritis, sarcoidosis, systemic mastocytosis
Malignant disease	Adenocarcinoma, carcinoid tumor, leiomyosarcoma, lymphoma, metastatic disease
Miscellaneous	Appendiceal disease, diverticular disease, nonsteroidal anti-inflammatory drug enteropathy, radiation enteritis, typhlitis

Fenkel JM, ed.
Quick Reference Dictionary for GI and Hepatology (pp 260-261).
© 2014 Taylor & Francis Group.

Etiology	Differential Diagnosis
Vascular	Behçet's disease, Henoch-Schönlein purpura, ischemia, polyarteritis nodosa, systemic lupus erythematosus, Wegener's granulomatosis

Human Immunodeficiency Virus in the GI Tract

Anatomical Location	Clinical Finding	Infectious Agent
Oropharynx	Thrush	*Candida*
	Hairy leukoplakia	Epstein-Barr virus
	Apthous ulcer	Herpes simplex virus
	Kaposi's sarcoma	Human herpes virus 8
	Palatal, glossal or gingival ulcers	*Cryptococcus* or histoplasma
Esophagus	Esophagitis	*Candida*, cytomegalovirus, herpes simplex virus
	Kaposi's sarcoma	Human herpes virus 8
	Lymphoma	Epstein-Barr virus
Stomach	Achlorydia	*Helicobacter pylori*
	Kaposi's sarcoma	Human herpes virus 8
	Lymphoma	Epstein-Barr virus
Pancreas	Pancreatitis	Pentamidine, didanosine, cytomegalovirus, mycobacterium avium complex, tuberculosis

Fenkel JM, ed.
Quick Reference Dictionary for GI and Hepatology (pp 262-264).
© 2014 Taylor & Francis Group.

Anatomical Location	Clinical Finding	Infectious Agent
Pancreas	Lymphoma	Epstein-Barr virus
	Kaposi's sarcoma	Human herpes virus 8
Liver	Viral hepatitis	Hepatitis B virus, hepatitis C virus
	Granulomatous hepatitis	*Mycobacterium avium* complex, coccidiomycosis, histoplasma
	Hepatic masses	Mycobacterium, peliosis hepatis, fungal infections, hepatocellular carcinoma, lymphoma
	Kaposi's sarcoma	Human herpes virus 8
	Papillary stenosis/ cholangiopathy	Cryptosporidiosis, cytomegalovirus, Kaposi's sarcoma
	Hepatic steatosis/ fulminant liver failure	Medications: nevirapine, idinavir, atazanavir
Small intestine	Diarrhea	Bacterial infections: *Salmonella, Shigella, Campylobacter, Mycobacterium avium* complex, small bowel bacterial overgrowth, tuberculosis
		Fungal infections: histoplasma, coccidiomycosis, penicilliosis, *Candida*

Anatomical Location	Clinical Finding	Infectious Agent
Small intestine		Protozoal infections: cryptosporidia, microsporidia, isospora, cyclospora
		Idiopathic: HIV enteropathy
		Viral: cytomegalovirus, herpes simplex virus, adenovirus
	Lymphoma	Epstein-Barr virus
	Kaposi's sarcoma	Human herpes virus 8
Colon	Colitis	Cytomegalovirus, *Clostridium difficile*
	Lymphoma	Epstein-Barr virus
	Kaposi's sarcoma	Human herpes virus 8
Rectum	Ulcers	Herpes simplex virus, HIV
	Condylomata accuminata	Human papilloma virus
	Kaposi's sarcoma	Human herpes virus 8
Peritoneum	Peritonitis	Coccidioidomycosis, tuberculosis

Screening and Surveillance for Colorectal Cancer

Several guidelines exist for colorectal cancer (CRC) screening. General and specific guidelines divided by risk group are discussed below. Screening is when you are doing a test in a patient with no previous history of CRC or adenomatous polyps. If the patient has had CRC or adenomatous polyps, then that patient is getting a surveillance procedure, not a screening one.

Abbreviations

AA: advanced adenoma (≥ 1 cm, or with villous component, or with high-grade or severe dysplasia)

ACG: American College of Gastroenterology

ACR: American College of Radiology

ACS: American Cancer Society

CRC: colorectal cancer

CT: computed tomography

DCBE: double contrast barium enema

DNA: deoxyribonucleic acid

FAP: familial adenomatous polyposis

FIT: fecal immunochemical test

FOBT: fecal occult blood test

Fenkel JM, ed.
Quick Reference Dictionary for GI and Hepatology (pp 265-271).
© *2014 Taylor & Francis Group.*

HNPCC: hereditary nonpolyposis colon cancer

NCCN: National Comprehensive Cancer Network

USMSTF: US Multi-Society Task Force on Colorectal Cancer

USPSTF: US Preventive Services Task Force

I. For Patients at Average Risk

- Screening should begin at age 50 years for both men and women.

- The ACG recommends screening start at age 45 years in African Americans.

- The USPSTF recommends cessation of routine screening in adults older than age 75 years.

- Methods of screening include tests that detect polyps and cancer, as well as tests that only detect cancer.

- CRC prevention tests detect polyps and cancer:
  - Colonoscopy
  - Flexible sigmoidoscopy
  - CT colonography
  - DCBE

- CRC detection tests detect only cancer:
  - FOBT
  - FIT
  - Stool DNA test

Table 19-1. Screening Methods for Patients at Average Risk

Test	Interval After Negative Test	Requires Bowel Prep?	Notes
Colonoscopy	Every 10 years	Yes	Preferred screening method by the ACG, ACS/USMSTF/ACR, and NCCN
Flexible sigmoidoscopy	Every 5 to 10 years ± FOBT every 3 years	Yes (partial)	Positive result → colonoscopy
CT colonography	Every 5 years	Yes	Polyps >5 mm → colonoscopy
DCBE	Every 5 years	Yes (partial)	No longer recommended by ACG, USPSTF, or NCCN
FOBT	Annually ± sigmoidoscopy every 5 years	No	Positive result → colonoscopy
FIT	Annually ± sigmoidoscopy every 5 years	No	Preferred cancer detection test by the ACG Positive result → colonoscopy
Stool DNA test	Uncertain—at least every 3 years	No	Positive result → colonoscopy

II. For Patients at Increased or High Risk

Table 19-2. Screening Strategy for Patients at Increased or High Risk

Risk Population	Recommendations	Screening Modality/Interval
Single first-degree relative with CRC or AA diagnosed at age 60 years or older	ACG, NCCN: screen as average risk ACS/USMSTF/ACR: start to screen at age 40 years	Screen as average risk using Table 1
Single first-degree relative with CRC or adenoma diagnosed at age younger than 60 years or 2 first-degree relatives with CRC or AA	Start to screen at age 40, or 10 years younger than the age of diagnosis of the youngest affected relative	Colonoscopy every 5 years
FAP	Start to screen at age 10 to 12 years	Annual colonoscopy or flexible sigmoidoscopy until colectomy deemed necessary

Risk Population	Recommendations	Screening Modality/Interval
HNPCC	Start to screen at age 20 to 25 years	Colonoscopy every 2 years until age 40 years, then annually
Inflammatory bowel disease	Start to screen 8 to 10 years after onset of symptoms	Colonoscopy with biopsies for dysplasia every 1 to 2 years

III. Surveillance for CRC After Polypectomy

Table 19-3. Surveillance for CRC Based on Prior Polyp Pathology

Finding on Colonoscopy	Screening Interval
Hyperplastic polyp(s)	Colonoscopy in 10 years
1 or 2 adenomas < 1 cm and with low-grade dysplasia	Colonoscopy in 5 to 10 years
3 to 10 adenomas or 1 AA	Colonoscopy in 3 years; if normal, or 1 to 2 low risk adenomas → 5 years
> 10 adenomas	< 3 years, as determined by clinician; consider possible underlying familial syndrome
Sessile adenoma removed piecemeal	2 to 6 months to verify complete removal, then surveillance interval determined by clinician
Inadequate bowel preparation and/or incomplete colonoscopy	Repeat examination

IV. SURVEILLANCE FOR CRC AFTER CANCER RESECTION

For patients who undergo resection with intent to cure or endoscopic resection of stage I cancer:

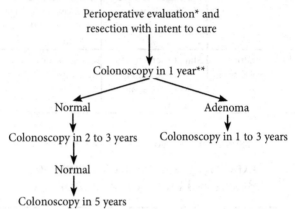

Perioperative evaluation* and resection with intent to cure

↓

Colonoscopy in 1 year**

Normal → Colonoscopy in 2 to 3 years → Normal → Colonoscopy in 5 years

Adenoma → Colonoscopy in 1 to 3 years

*Patients should have perioperative evaluation for synchronous lesions either by colonoscopy, CT colonography, or DBCE in the case of obstructing CRC.

**Examination of the rectum to evaluate for local recurrence after low anterior resection of rectal cancer can be performed every 3 to 6 month for the first 2 to 3 years. This is in addition to surveillance colonoscopy.

BIBLIOGRAPHY

Burt R, Barthel J, Dunn K, et al. NCCN clinical practice guidelines in oncology. Colorectal cancer screening. J Natl Compr Canc Netw. 2010;8:8-61.

Levin B, Lieberman DA, McFarland B, et al. Screening and surveillance for the early detection of colorectal cancer and adenomatous polyps, 2008: a joint guideline from the American Cancer Society, the US Multi-Society Task Force on Colorectal Cancer, and the American College of Radiology. *CA Cancer J Clin.* 2008;58:130-160.

Rex D, Johnson D, Anderson J, et al. American College of Gastroenterology Guidelines for colorectal cancer screening 2008. *Am J Gastroenterol.* 2009;104:739-750.

U.S. Preventive Services Task Force. Screening for colorectal cancer: US Preventive Services Task Force recommendation statement. *Ann Intern Med.* 2008;149:627-637.

Winawer SJ, Zauber AG, Fletcher RH, et al. Guidelines for colonoscopy surveillance after polypectomy: a consensus update by the US Multi-Society Task Force on Colorectal Cancer and the American Cancer Society. *Gastroenterology.* 2006;130:1872-1885.

Classification of GI Bleeding

- Overt: Active, ongoing upper or lower GI bleeding presenting as hematochezia, melena, or hematemesis with an identifiable source located on standard endoscopic or radiologic methods.

- Occult: Active GI blood loss in the absence of obvious hemorrhage (hemoccult positive) with an identifiable cause detected using standard endoscopic or radiologic methods.

- Obscure: Recurrent GI bleeding in the absence of an identifiable cause found using standard endoscopic or radiologic methods.

  ○ Obscure-overt: Overt bleeding with a concurrent active hemoglobin drop, often accompanied by signs of hypovolemic shock, without an identifiable cause on upper or lower endoscopy and appropriate radiologic tests.

  ○ Obscure-occult: The absence of overt bleeding with evidence of microscopic (hemoccult) positive stool, without an identifiable cause on upper or lower endoscopy and appropriate radiologic tests. This category usually includes iron-deficiency anemia.

Fenkel JM, ed.
Quick Reference Dictionary for GI and Hepatology (pp 272).
© 2014 Taylor & Francis Group.

Classification of Irritable Bowel Syndrome

Irritable bowel syndrome (IBS) is a common condition encountered in a gastroenterology practice. Unfortunately, no specific diagnostic test exists to determine whether a patient has IBS. As such, a conference of experts helped craft consensus criteria for diagnosing functional gastrointestinal disorders, such as IBS. These criteria are known as the Rome III criteria and are accessible online at www.romecriteria.org/assets/pdf/19_RomeIII_apA_885-898.pdf.

The diagnostic criteria for IBS are the following:

- Recurrent abdominal pain or discomfort at least 3 days per month in the past 3 months, with symptom onset at least 6 months prior, associated with 2 or more of the following:

  ○ Improvement with defecation.

  ○ Onset associated with a change in frequency of stool.

  ○ Onset associated with a change in form (appearance) of stool.

- Patients with IBS can be further classified into subgroups based on their stool form, using the Bristol Stool Form (BSF) scale.

Fenkel JM, ed.
Quick Reference Dictionary for GI and Hepatology (pp 273-274).
© 2014 Taylor & Francis Group.

BSF Scale

Type	Description
1	Separate hard lumps like nuts
2	Sausage shaped but lumpy
3	Like a sausage but with cracks on its surface
4	Like a sausage or snake, smooth and soft
5	Soft blobs with clear-cut edges
6	Fluffy pieces with ragged edges, a mushy stool
7	Watery, no solid pieces

Subgroups of IBS According to Rome III Criteria

1. IBS with constipation (IBS-C): BSF scale score of 1 or 2 in 25% or more of stools and BSF scale score of 6 or 7 in less than 25% of stools.

2. IBS with diarrhea (IBS-D): BSF scale score of 6 or 7 in 25% or more of stools and BSF scale score of 1 or 2 in less than 25% of stools.

3. Mixed IBS (IBS-M): BSF scale score of 1 or 2 in 25% or more of stools and BSF scale score of 6 or 7 in 25% or more of stools.

4. Unsubtyped IBS (IBS-U): insufficient abnormality of stool consistency to meet criteria for any of the subgroups.

Bibliography

Ersyd A, Posserud I, Abrahamsson H, Simrén M. Subtyping the irritable bowel syndrome by predominant bowel habit: Rome II versus Rome III. *Aliment Pharmacol Ther.* 2007;26:953-961.

Lewis SJ, Heaton KW. Stool form scale as a useful guide to intestinal transit time. *Scand J Gastroenterol.* 1997; 32:920-924.

Rome III Criteria. http://romecriteria.org/assets/pdf/19_RomeIII_apA_885-898.pdf. Accessed February 12, 2013.

Velasco B, Fisher, R. Irritable bowel syndrome. *Bope & Kellerman: Conn's Current Therapy.* 1st ed. New York: Saunders; 2012:544-546.

Gluten-Free Foods and Sample Daily Diet for Patients With Celiac Disease

NATURALLY OCCURRING GLUTEN-FREE FOODS[a]

Proteins	Vegetables	Grains	Fruits	Dairy
Steak	All vegetables	Rice (and wild rice)	All fruits	Milk
Chicken		Corn		Cheese
Turkey		Quinoa		Butter
Bacon		Millet		Yogurt
Duck		Amaranth		
Fish		Buckwheat		
Tofu		Sorghum		
Beans		Soy		
Nuts/seeds		Tapioca		
Nutbutters				

[a]This list is just a representation of the basic gluten-free foods available and does not illustrate the entire spectrum or any of the processed foods. In addition, individuals who need to consume gluten-free foods should always check the ingredients list before eating. In their raw form, these products should not contain gluten; however, it will often be added in more processed versions.

Fenkel JM, ed.
Quick Reference Dictionary for GI and Hepatology (pp 275-278).
© 2014 Taylor & Francis Group.

SAMPLE DAILY DIET FOR
PATIENTS WITH CELIAC DISEASE

Breakfast	Lunch/Dinner	Snacks	Dessert
Gluten-free cereals with milk	Sandwich on gluten-free bread or lettuce wrap	Melted cheese over chips	Fruit
Egg (any way you like it!)	Gluten-free soups	Celery with peanut butter or cream cheese	Crème brule
Oatmeal (gluten-free oats only)	Baked potato	Nuts	Maca-roons
Yogurt	Roast chicken (any kind of meat or poultry), rice, and vegetables	Veggies and bean dip	Flan
Fruit	Gluten-free pasta with tomato sauce or pesto and vegetables	Chips with salsa or guacamole	Sorbet
Smoothies	Beans and rice	Rice cake with peanut butter or apple butter	Gelato (no cookie flavors)

Breakfast	Lunch/Dinner	Snacks	Dessert
Gluten-free toast with jam, nut butter, cream cheese, or butter	Salads with or without meat	Popcorn	Gluten-free rice crispy treats
Grits	Quesadillas on corn tortillas, corn tacos, or tostadas on corn tortillas	Yogurt with gluten-free granola	Popsicles
	Tuna/chicken salad	Cheese	
	Stir-fries	Fruit	
		Snack bars	
		Hard boiled egg	

NATIONAL CELIAC DISEASE SUPPORT GROUPS

Celiac Disease Foundation

20350 Ventura Blvd, Suite 240

Woodland Hills, CA 91364

Phone: (818) 716-1513

Website: www.celiac.org

National Foundation for Celiac Awareness
124 South Maple St
Ambler, PA 19002
Phone: (215) 325-1306
Website: www.celiaccentral.org

Gluten Intolerance Group
31214 124th Ave SE
Auburn, WA 98092
Phone: (253) 833-6655
Website: www.gluten.net

Celiac Support Association
P.O. Box 31700
Omaha, NE 68131-0700
Phone: (877) 272-4272
Phone: (402) 558-0600
Website: www.csaceliacs.info

Pancreaticobiliary

Scoring of Acute Pancreatitis

Acute pancreatitis is a disease that can have significant morbidity and mortality. Many efforts have been made to help predict its severity by developing scoring systems, and models have taken place over the past 15 to 20 years. No one system is perfect, but they still have value, particularly by aiding clinicians in admitting patients to intensive care if they are predicted to have higher mortality rate. One of the most common classification systems used by most gastroenterologists is based on criteria developed at a symposium in Atlanta, Georgia, in 1992, now called the Atlanta Criteria. It differentiates acute pancreatitis into mild and severe cases. It requires knowledge of two other scoring systems, Ranson's criteria and the Acute Physiology and Chronic Health Examination (APACHE II) score, which are detailed below.

ATLANTA CRITERIA

- Mild pancreatitis: Pancreatitis associated with minimal organ dysfunction and an uneventful recovery.

- Severe (necrotizing) pancreatitis: Any of the following 4 options:

  ○ Ranson's score ≥ 3

  ○ APACHE II score ≥ 8

  ○ Organ failure (includes GI bleeding and renal, respiratory, or circulatory failure):

Fenkel JM, ed.
Quick Reference Dictionary for GI and Hepatology (pp 280-284).
© 2014 Taylor & Francis Group.

- Circulatory: systolic blood pressure < 90 mm Hg
- Respiratory: $PaO_2 \leq 60$ mm Hg
- Renal: serum creatinine > 2 mg/dL
- GI bleeding: > 500 mL within 24 hour
  - Local complications, such as pancreatic pseudocyst, necrosis, or abscess

RANSON'S CRITERIA

- 11 variables (5 on admission, 6 after 48 hours) with 1 point awarded for each positive criterion.

- A score from 0 to 2 predicts a mortality rate of < 3%, a score of 3 to 4 predicts a mortality rate of 11% to 15%, and a score of > 5 predicts a mortality rate of 40%.

RANSON'S CRITERIA

Ranson's Criteria for Pancreatitis	1 point for every YES
At admission...	
Is age older than 55 years?	
Is white blood cell count > 16,000 cells/mm^3?	
Is blood glucose > 200 mg/dL?	
Is lactate dehydrogenase > 350 IU/L?	
Is aspartate aminotransferase > 250?	
After 48 hours...	
Does hematocrit decrease by > 10%?	
Does blood urea nitrogen (BUN) increase by > 5 mg/dL?	
Does calcium decrease to < 8 mg/dL?	
Does PaO_2 decrease to < 60 mm Hg?	
Is the base deficit (24-HCO_3) > 4 mEq/L?	
Is the estimated fluid sequestration > 6 L?	

APACHE II Score

- Includes 12 variables from admission only, with added complexity for the presence of chronic disease and age.

- Was originally designed to predict intensive care unit mortality.

- A score ≥ 8 predicts an 11% to 18% mortality rate.

- A score < 8 predicts a 4% mortality rate.

- Online calculators are available to help calculate the score, and this complexity limits common practice. The American Gastroenterological Association recommends using an APACHE II score ≥ 8 to predict severe disease.

- Variables include the following:
  - Rectal temperature
  - Mean arterial blood pressure
  - Heart rate
  - Respiratory rate
  - A-a gradient or pulse oximetry
  - Arterial pH or HCO_3
  - Sodium
  - Potassium
  - Creatinine
  - Hematocrit
  - White blood cell count
  - Glasgow Coma score
  - Age
  - Presence of chronic disease

Other Scoring Systems

Computed Tomography (CT) Severity Score (Balthazar Score)

- Uses CT scan findings to predict severity of clinical course.

- Score has 2 components:
  - Necrosis percentage
  - Grading of inflammation and fluid collections
- Higher scores predict a greater likelihood of death, need for necrosectomy, and longer hospital stays.

BISAP Score

- A bedside tool to grade severity during the first 24 hours of patient care.
- Score ranges from 0 to 5:
  - Score of 0 to 2 predicts a mortality rate of < 2%.
  - Score of 3 to 5 predicts a mortality rate of > 15%.
- B = BUN > 25 mg/dL
- I = impaired mental status
- S = presence of systemic inflammatory response syndrome
- A = age > 60 years
- P = pleural effusion

Systemic Inflammatory Response Syndrome (SIRS) Score

- Calculates the presence or absence of SIRS on admission and at 24 and 48 hours after admission.
- Patients with SIRS persistent throughout admission had the highest mortality rate (27%) compared with those who did not have persistent SIRS (3% mortality).
- SIRS is defined by possessing 2 of the following 4 criteria:
  - Pulse > 90
  - Respiratory rate > 20 or PaO_2 < 32 mm Hg
  - Temperature > 38°C or < 36°C
  - White blood cell count > 12,000 or < 4000

BIBLIOGRAPHY

Banks PA, Freeman ML; and the Practice Parameters Committee of the American College of Gastroenterology. Practice guidelines in acute pancreatitis. *Am J Gastroenterol.* 2006;101:2379-2400.

Bradley EL 3rd. A clinically based classification system for acute pancreatitis. Summary of the International Symposium on Acute Pancreatitis, Atlanta, Ga, September 11 through 13, 1992. *Arch Surg.* 1993;128:586-590.

Buter A, Imrie CW, Carter CR, Evans S, McKay CJ. Dynamic nature of early organ dysfunction determines outcome in acute pancreatitis. *Br J Surg.* 2002;89:298-302.

Tenner S, Steinberg WM. Acute pancreatitis. In: Feldman M, Friedman LS, Brandt LJ, eds. *Sleisenger and Fordtran's Gastrointestinal and Liver Disease.* 9th ed. Philadelphia: Elsevier; 2010:959-976.

Wu BU, Johannes RS, Sun X, Tabak Y, Conwell DL, Banks PA. The early prediction of mortality in acute pancreatitis: a large population-based study. *Gut.* 2008;57:1698-1703.

Differential Diagnosis of a Pancreatic Mass

I. Solid Pancreatic Mass

Type of Solid Mass	Notes
PDA	90% of pancreatic neoplasms
	Poor prognosis
	Surgical resection is potentially curative
Pancreatic lymphoma	< 1% of pancreatic neoplasms
	Difficult to differentiate from PDA; requires biopsy
	Better prognosis than PDA; responds to chemotherapy with or without surgery
Pancreatic neuroendocrine tumor	3% of pancreatic neoplasms
	Insulinoma, gastrinoma, glucagonoma, VIPoma, and somatostatinoma
	May require EUS or nuclear imaging for localization

Fenkel JM, ed.
Quick Reference Dictionary for GI and Hepatology (pp 285-289).
© 2014 Taylor & Francis Group.

Type of Solid Mass	Notes
Mass-forming chronic pancreatitis	Most often in alcoholics, also genetic syndromes
	Chronic pancreatitis is risk factor for PDA
Autoimmune pancreatitis	Rare autoimmune disorder with recurrent episodes of pancreatitis
	Elevated IgG4, positive ANA, and biopsy can help differentiate from PDA
	Responsive to steroids
Metastasis from other primary cancer	Rare
	Includes cancer of the lung, breast, kidney, stomach, melanoma, HCC, thyroid, and osteoscarcoma
	Rarely discovered before primary cancer detected

PDA, pancreatic ductal adenocarcinoma; EUS, endoscopic ultrasound; ANA, antinuclear antibody; HCC, hepatocellular carcinoma; VIP, vasoactive intestinal peptide.

II. Cystic Pancreatic Mass

- Cystic neoplasms represent less than 10% of pancreatic neoplasms.

- Symptomatic masses of any etiology can be treated with surgical resection.

- Fine-needle aspiration of the cyst fluid with or without wall by EUS or a percutaneous approach, endoscopic retrograde cholangiopancreatography, and surveillance imaging can be used to determine the diagnosis and malignant potential.

Type of Cystic Mass	Notes/Features	Cyst Fluid Amylase	Cyst Fluid CEA	Malignant Potential
Pancreatic pseudocyst	90+% of cysts	↑	↓	No
	History of acute or chronic pancreatitis			
	Unlilocular, with a thick wall			
	M > F			
Serous cystadenoma	Multilocular	↓	↓	No
	Central scar on CT or MRI			
	F > M			
MCN	One cyst, often with thick walls and septations	↓	↑	Yes
	F > M			
	Mucin-rich fluid			
Intraductal papillary mucinous neoplasm	Pancreatic duct dilatation	↑	↑	Yes
	Main duct or branch duct subtypes			
Solid pseudopapillary neoplasm	Mixed solid mass with fluid	↓	↓	Yes
	F > M			
	Necrotic debris in cyst			

Type of Cystic Mass	Notes/Features	Cyst Fluid Amylase	Cyst Fluid CEA	Malignant Potential
Acinar-cell cystadeno-carcinoma	Variable appearance	↑/↓	↑	Yes
	M > F			
Cystic endo-crine neo-plasm	Variable appearance	↓	↓	Yes, similar to solid NET
	M = F			
PDA with cys-tic degen-eration	Mass with localized fluid collection	↓	↑	This is malignant
	M > F			
	Adeno-carcinoma on FNA cytology			

CEA, carcinoembryonic antigen; M, male; F, female; MCN, mucinous cystic neoplasm; NET, neuroendocrine tumor; PDA, pancreatic ductal adenocarcinoma; FNA, fine needle aspiration.

BIBLIOGRAPHY

Brugge WR, Lauwers GY, Sahani D, Fernandez-del Castillo C, Warshaw AL. Cystic neoplasms of the pancreas. *N Engl J Med.* 2004;351:1218-1226.

Finkelberg DL, Sahani D, Deshpande V, Brugge WR. Autoimmune pancreatitis. *N Engl J Med.* 2006;355:2670-2676.

Hong SK, Loren DE, Rogart JN, et al. Targeted cyst wall puncture and aspiration during EUS-FNA increases the diagnostic yield of premalignant and malignant pancreatic cysts. *Gastrointest Endosc.* 2012;75:775-782.

Luo G, Jin C, Fu D, Long J, Yang F, Ni Q. Primary pancreatic lymphoma. *Tumori.* 2009;95:156-159.

Scatarige JC, Horton KM, Sheth S, Fishman EK. Pancreatic parenchymal metastases: observations on helical CT. *AJR Am J Roentgenol.* 2001;176:695-699.

Sheiman J. Cystic lesions of the pancreas. *Gastroenterology.* 2005;128:463-469.

Stevens T, Conwell DL. Pancreatic neoplasms. Cleveland Clinic Center for Continuing Education. http://www.clevelandclinicmeded.com/medicalpubs/diseasemanagement/gastroenterology/pancreatic-neoplasms/. Published August 1, 2010. Accessed March 5, 2012.

Yoon WJ, Brugge WR. Pancreatic cystic neoplasms: diagnosis and management. *Gastroenterol Clin N Am.* 2012;41:103-118.

Types of Sphincter of Oddi Dysfunction

Type of SOD	Biliary-Type Pain	Abnormal Liver Tests[a]	Abnormal Imaging[b]	Manometry Before Endoscopic Sphincterotomy?
1	Yes	Yes	Yes	No
2	Yes	Must have abnormal liver tests or abnormal imaging as above	Must have abnormal liver tests or abnormal imaging as above	Yes
3	Yes	No	No	Yes

SOD, sphincter of Oddi; ERCP, endoscopic retrograde cholangiopancreatography; CBD, common bile duct.

[a]AST, ALT, or AlkPhos more than twice normal levels that are documented on 2 or more occasions.

[b]Delayed draining of ERCP contrast for more than 45 minutes or dilated CBD (more than 10 mm on cholangiography or more than 12 mm on ultrasound).

Fenkel JM, ed.
Quick Reference Dictionary for GI and Hepatology (pp 290-291).
© 2014 Taylor & Francis Group.

BIBLIOGRAPHY

Bistritz L, Bai VG. Sphincter of Oddi dysfunction: managing the patient with chronic biliary pain. *World J Gastroenterol.* 2006;12:3793-3802.

Sgouros SN, Pereira SP. Systematic review: sphincter of Oddi dysfunction—non-invasive diagnostic methods and long-term outcome after endoscopic sphincterotomy. *Aliment Pharmacol Ther.* 2006;24:237-246.

Sherman S, Lehman GA. Sphincter of Oddi dysfunction: diagnosis and treatment. *JOP* 2001;2:382-400.

Types of Gallstones

Gallstones are small, solid, rock-like substances that sometimes form in the gallbladder or bile ducts. Cholelithiasis (the presence of gallstones) is often asymptomatic but can lead to significant morbidity if the stones migrate out of the gallbladder and obstruct the cystic duct or common bile duct. There are 2 main types of gallstones: cholesterol and pigment. Pigment stones can be further subdivided into black or brown. Occasionally, a combination of cholesterol and pigment stones occurs and is referred to as a mixed stone.

1. Cholesterol stones

   ○ *Epidemiology:* Account for 80% of gallstones in the United States; are most prevalent in Western populations; and have the highest world prevalence among the Pima Indians.

   ○ *Risk factors:* Obesity, advanced age, female sex, estrogen exposure (such as with oral contraceptive use or pregnancy), rapid weight loss or prolonged fasting, decreased gallbladder motility, syndromes resulting in hyperlipidemia, and rare inborn errors of bile acid metabolism.

   ○ *Pathogenesis:* Bile consists of a mixture of cholesterol, bile acids, and lecithin (a phospholipid). When the relative proportion of cholesterol is high due to the acquired risk factors referred to above or to genetic factors (as seen

Fenkel JM, ed.
Quick Reference Dictionary for GI and Hepatology (pp 292-294).
© 2014 Taylor & Francis Group.

in Pima Indians), cholesterol can precipitate out. It then forms crystals (microlithiasis) that interact with calcium salts and mucus, forming macroscopic gallstones.

2. Pigment stones

Pigment stones are less common than cholesterol stones and are predominately seen in non-Western populations. There are two types—black and brown—that have different risk factors and pathogenesis, but both are mostly composed of bilirubin and calcium salts.

○ Black pigment stones

- *Epidemiology:* Most commonly seen in conditions causing excess unconjugated bilirubin levels, such as in chronic hemolytic diseases, but can develop in patients with cirrhosis, as well as those receiving total parenteral nutrition.

- *Pathogenesis:* When the concentration of unconjugated bilirubin in bile becomes high, it can bind with calcium to form insoluble salts, leading to the development of black pigment stones. These stones usually develop in the gallbladder.

○ Brown pigment stones

- *Epidemiology:* Most often associated with biliary tract infections, including *Escherichia coli, Ascaris lumbricoides,* or *Opisthorchis sinensis* (also known as "liver fluke").

- *Pathogenesis:* Form in the presence of bacterial enzymes, which hydrolyze bilirubin and lecithin. The hydrolysis of bilirubin forms unconjugated bilirubin, which combines with calcium to form insoluble salts. In addition, the hydrolysis of lecithin leads to the formation of calcium palmitate, which combines with the calcium bilirubinate to form a brown pigment stone. These stones usually present in the intrahepatic or extrahepatic bile ducts.

BIBLIOGRAPHY

Bajwa N, Bajwa R, Ghumman A, Agrawal RM. The Gallstone Story: Pathogenesis and Epidemiology. *Practical Gastroenterology*. 2010;34:11-23.

Financial Disclosures

Dr. Jennifer Au has not disclosed any relevant financial relationships.

Dr. Alia Dadabhai has no financial or proprietary interest in the materials presented herein.

Dr. Jonathan M. Fenkel is a consultant for Vertex Pharamaceuticals, Idenix Pharmaceuticals, Gilead Pharmaceuticals, and Janssen Therapeutics.

Dr. Jessica Jackson has not disclosed any relevant financial relationships.

Annsley Klehr has no financial or proprietary interest in the materials presented herein.

Dr. Steven Krawitz has no financial or proprietary interest in the materials presented herein.

Dr. Christina Lindenmeyer has no financial or proprietary interest in the materials presented herein.

Dr. Aaron Mendelson has no financial or proprietary interest in the materials presented herein.

Dr. Anastasia Shnitser has no financial or proprietary interest in the materials presented herein.

Dr. Colin Smith has no financial or proprietary interest in the materials presented herein.

Dr. Joanna Tolin has no financial or proprietary interest in the materials presented herein.